Regaining the Power of Youth
• • • • • • • • • • • • • •

at Any Age

Regaining the Power of Youth

at Any Age

KENNETH H. COOPER, M.D., M.P.H.

Publishers Since 1798

THOMAS NELSON PUBLISHERS

Nashville

Published in Nashville, Tennessee, by Thomas Nelson, Inc.

The Bible version used in this publication is THE NEW KING JAMES VERSION. Copyright © 1979, 1980, 1982, 1990, Thomas Nelson, Inc.

Library of Congress Cataloging-in-Publication Data

Cooper, Kenneth H.
   Regaining the power of youth at any age / Kenneth H. Cooper.
     p.   cm.
   ISBN 0-7852-7142-2 (hc)
    1. Longevity—Popular works. 2. Health—Popular works. 3. Physical fitness—Popular works. I. Title.
   RA776.75.C665 1998
   613—dc21   98-45029
                                                CIP

Printed in the United States of America.

1 2 3 4 5 6 BVG 03 02 01 00 99 98

To the family,
both in the United States and
elsewhere around the world.
Though under seige,
this relationship is still
a great source of hope for our future—
and for helping us rediscover
the Power of Youth in our lives.

Acknowledgments

We live in an age when the focus of many health-oriented books is self-centered and narcissistic. We are told that the most important thing in life is to achieve and maintain a youthful look—and the skills of plastic surgeons, dermatologists, and fitness trainers are mobilized to this end.

The logical conclusion of this line of reasoning is that true happiness is possible only if we can maintain some illusion of agelessness, or even immortality. An underlying assumption seems to be that—contrary to all we have been taught about true beauty and values being on the inside—outward appearance is all that counts.

My more than forty years of medical practice and research in the science of physical fitness and preventive medicine—not to mention my basic life experience—have convinced me that just the opposite is true. A youthful, healthy body is important, but only to the extent that it can prepare us for more vigorous action at work, at home, and in our relationships, especially family relationships.

Certainly, a benefit of having a youthful body and nimble mind is that you are more likely to feel better about yourself. But this enhanced sense of self-esteem depends more on an inner transformation of your expectations than it does on outward appearance.

In *Regaining the Power of Youth at Any Age,* my objective has been to show you the way—through my own research and experience, as well as that of patients and colleagues—to this personal transformation. In many cases, actual names have been used in the text. But, as with previous books, I've also chosen to disguise the identity of those involved in various case studies to protect confidential patient and personal information. I often try to make this practice clear by enclosing the first reference to a changed identity in quotation marks.

In exploring the latest scientific frontiers of personal vigor, stamina, and strength, I've relied on the help of a host of other professionals, including:

- My professional literary collaborator, William Proctor. Bill has worked with me since 1980. *Regaining the Power of Youth at Any Age,* our eleventh project, is in many respects the culmination of all that has gone before.
- My literary agent, Herbert M. Katz, who has worked with me, either as editor or agent, for more than thirty years. Herb and his colleague and wife, Nancy Katz, have been instrumental in representing my business interests and also in establishing a strong international presence for many of my books.
- My secretary and administrative assistant, Harriet Guthrie, who has helped keep my schedule in order and my life sane for almost twenty years. Harriet retired just as this book was going to press, and I certainly wish her and her husband, Bill, well in this next phase of their lives.
- My supportive family, especially my wife, Millie, who, through her vibrant, energetic example, has taught me more than she will ever know about the true meaning of the power of youth.
- The highly effective publishing and editing team at Thomas Nelson. Over the past six years, these top-notch executives, editors, and administrators have graciously provided me with the platform to spread the gospel of preventive medicine.

Now, without further delay, let's see what we can learn about the real meaning of *Regaining the Power of Youth at Any Age.*

Part 1

....

THE POWER OF YOUTH AT ANY AGE

1
• • • • • • • • • • • • • •

Targeting:
Your Path to the Power of Youth

One of my greatest weaknesses is that the older I get, the more likely I am to give in to the temptation to test my physical and emotional limits.

I may tell you that I want to push my personal envelope because as a sixty-seven-year-old preventive medicine specialist, I need to explore just how far the aging body and mind can go. But in my secret heart of hearts there's more involved than mere medical experimentation. *Much, much more*, I mused as I sat astride a mountain bike atop 10,200-foot Spruce Saddle in the shadow of Grouse Mountain, gazing down on the village of Beaver Creek, Colorado, 2,100 feet below.

I had talked my friend and professional writer, Bill Proctor, into joining me, and I was feeling quite confident because the two of us had biked down this mountain the year before. What I didn't know was that a new route we had chosen harbored some challenges that we weren't quite prepared for.

On the previous occasion, we had stuck to a dirt access road, which—though rough as a washboard and full of sharp curves, rocks, and ditches—had been manageable. The narrow trail we now found ourselves on was a different matter entirely.

This two-mile trek was only one or two feet wide. Pockmarked by sharp mini-boulders and abrupt ditches, it featured hairpin turns to end all hairpin turns. We later learned the trail had been designated one of the more difficult routes and was used by competitive bikers for cross-country races.

Because we were completely unfamiliar with the terrain, we kept making crucial mistakes. We'd shift into a low gear and accelerate as we climbed a slight rise only to find ourselves plunging at excessive speeds almost straight down after we reached a crest. To make matters worse, the trail often slanted toward the edge of the mountain. If we weren't careful, our bikes could creep over that edge and we'd find ourselves tumbling onto the steep, rocky mountainside, with no guarantee where our descent might end.

As we navigated these tight turns and steep descents, we were discovering that the skills required to manipulate the brakes and otherwise maneuver the bikes on such a treacherous path were a little beyond us. When we signed the release that's required when you rent a bike to use on these trails, we had to indicate whether we were classified as *novice*, *intermediate*, *advanced*, or *expert*. Bill had suggested that perhaps we should create another category—*sub-novice*. But I confidently advised him, "No, no, check *intermediate*. We're definitely *intermediate*."

I was having second thoughts about that choice.

Take the brakes, for instance. I knew that a prime rule of downhill mountain biking is to use the back brake more than the front brake. The reason: if a cyclist is whizzing pell-mell down a slope and hits only the front brake, the front wheel will certainly stop rotating. Then, most likely, *he'll* begin rotating as the back wheel bucks up and he flips head over heels, somersaulting down the mountain.

On this particular trail, a different braking technique was required, one that had somehow slipped my mind. Specifically, when headed down a rough, steep slope, a mountain biker does have to rely primarily on the back brake. But he must also pump the front brake in

4

order to keep the bike stable as he skids along. Because I was using the back brake almost exclusively, my bike started to fishtail. I had to stop several times on the sharpest turns to avoid tipping over or careening off the trail entirely.

Another problem was the rented bikes. Although we were both accustomed to using bikes without shock absorbers, this time we had chosen models with shocks—one each on both the front and back wheels for my bike, and one on the front for Bill's. The main idea was to make the ride more comfortable. Also, experienced mountain bikers always use shocks to cushion the bone-rattling impact of the ride on hands, arms, and bottom. But the combination of the braking demands and the unaccustomed shock absorbers gave me a disturbingly unstable, out-of-control feeling as we bounced and skidded down the mountain.

I was worried about Bill, who was bumping along a few feet behind me. *Poor Bill*, I thought. *He could hurt himself. I can just see him laid up in a hospital bed, his legs in traction. How will I explain this to his wife? Will we ever finish this power of youth book? Not only that, Bill is fifty-six years old. A serious injury might make it impossible for him to regain what little youth he has left!*

Just then I noticed that a particularly challenging hairpin turn was looming ahead, so I decided to improvise. A barely discernible path seemed to lead off the main trail and then back to it. This path would enable me to avoid the upcoming turn and perhaps assert more control over my bike. So I swerved off and headed down the alternate route.

Unfortunately, I did a bad job of anticipating my own speed and the severe angle of the slope, not to mention the near-impossibility of negotiating a successful turn to reenter the main trail. I sailed right across the trail and shot up into the air, at which point my bike and I parted company.

Bill, who had, more wisely, chosen to stay on the trail and take his chances with the hairpin turn, watched the spectacle with some awe.

"You were suspended in air, with arms spread out like wings," he told me later. "All I could think of was, 'It's a bird, it's a plane, it's Superdoc!'"

But Bill's amazement turned into real worry when I disappeared headfirst into some high grass and failed to reappear for several seconds. Finally, I did emerge—but with a few hard-earned lessons now at the top of my mind.

First of all, I became even more of a believer in protective helmets than in the past. What Bill didn't see was that I had crashed headlong into a large rock. Without a helmet, I would have suffered a concussion or something much worse. The reason that I was so slow to get up was that the blow to my head had actually dazed me for a few seconds.

Second, the accident confirmed for me the importance of doing specificity training—or what's called *targeting* in this book—to build bones and muscles as we get older.

I had landed heavily on my left shoulder. My collarbone was hurting, and I immediately tested it gingerly to be sure nothing was broken. All my bones were okay. The main reason, I'm convinced, was that a number of years before, I had embarked on a "striking," or bone-building, program of the type I'm advocating in this book. At my age, if I had failed to stick to a regimen that maintains bone density, I would be in the position of most people my age, having a skeletal structure that was relatively brittle and certainly too weak to have withstood the impact of that fall.

Finally, and perhaps most important, I was reminded once again of the importance of knowing my limits as I grow older.

There was nothing wrong with my going out for a rigorous mountain-biking adventure at age sixty-seven because I've had considerable experience using these vehicles on the Colorado terrain. Also, I knew that I had done adequate strength and aerobic training to meet most of the demands of such an outing.

But I had pushed my personal envelope a little too far in this situation. I should have slowed down and been more careful because I was riding an unfamiliar bike on an unfamiliar trail. Instead, I took some unnecessary risks. Fortunately, I escaped serious injury— though I must admit I needed some aspirin that night to relieve soreness in my left shoulder and neck!

This incident reminds me that as I grow older, I must become more vigilant about what's needed to maintain a high level of energy and strength. Yet my experience just scratches the surface of what it means to regain the power of youth at my age or yours. The search for the power of youth is an ongoing quest—which will become evident as we explore this new frontier of total, age-sensitive fitness in the following pages.

THE QUEST FOR THE POWER OF YOUTH

What is the power of youth?

The power of youth is vigor. It's the power of boundless energy and stamina; the power of emotional resilience and optimism; the power of agile reasoning, creative thinking, and comprehensive memory.

When we are young, this power may infuse us with a sense of invulnerability, even immortality. But as we grow older, and especially as we enter the middle years of life, we often find that our early feelings of vigor fade and then disappear altogether. Take a moment to test yourself:

- Do you frequently feel that you are "running on empty"?
- Are you frazzled more than once a week as you juggle the demands of family, child rearing, and work?
- Do you seem to be growing more distractible and forgetful?
- As you encounter more aches, pains, and stiffness, do you ever worry that you are getting old before your time?
- Is your typical response to the demands of daily life characterized by early-onset fatigue, a general sense of boredom, or mind-numbing burnout?

Such symptoms are prevalent among most mature age-groups in our society, from young middle-agers in their thirties, to the more than seventy-eight million baby boomers, four million of whom have already turned fifty, to the burgeoning ranks of older adults. In short, increasing numbers of people are finding that they are incapable of working to their maximum capacity, relating effectively to others, or otherwise achieving their full potential in life, primarily because they simply don't have the "get-up-and-go" to meet their daily responsibilities.

My diagnosis of this pervasive, age-related loss of vigor may be described by the general term *youth drain*. But the underlying cause of the condition is not simply the process of human aging. Rather, youth drain arises from a prolonged exposure over years to a number of negative outside forces, which buffet and batter us into chronic physical fatigue, mental dullness, and eventually poor health.

SOME MAJOR CAUSES OF YOUTH DRAIN
AND THE TARGETING RESPONSE

As we age, we steadily lose the power of youth not because of the passage of years, but rather because of a failure to respond to and overcome such factors as:

- nagging, recurrent health complaints
- feelings of no longer competing at a high level
- tension caused by time pressures
- the punishing emotional and physical effects of too much unwanted travel, particularly business travel
- financial worries
- the unexpected effects of menopause—both male and female
- frustrations with child rearing
- exhaustion from technology and information overload
- wrong expectations about health and the aging process

We'll deal in some detail with these causes of youth drain in Chapter 4. But first, let me introduce you to the fundamental strategy that I've found to be the most effective way to overcome most causes of youth drain—and to recapture the power of youth.

Sometimes, when a disease or infection is involved, the only reasonable response is medication or another procedure wholly controlled by a qualified physician. But many times a specific health challenge can be handled with a specific preventive measure that involves self-diagnosis and sometimes even self-treatment—an approach that I call *targeting*. Targeting is a scientifically proven strategy of self-assessment and self-treatment that features the application of specific fitness, diet, and psychological techniques to particular health concerns. Targeting also encompasses special skills that can help patients collaborate effectively with their physicians.

This definition has many practical applications, which are inserted throughout the book as sidebars. These sidebar boxes contain a variety of guidelines and recommendations for developing your own targeting strategies with exercise, food, nutritional supplements, psychological ploys, spiritual disciplines, and medical prescriptions or procedures.

To help you better understand how these targeting techniques may be employed, I've provided them with labels:

- *quick fix*, a psychological or fitness tactic to banish a temporary ache or pain
- *stamina strategy*, an exercise to improve a particular kind of physical endurance or strength
- *eye-opener*, a routine to promote alertness early in the day
- *pick-me-up*, a regimen to gain an infusion of energy later in the day
- *stopgap*, a short workout to maintain a minimal level of conditioning when you lack time for a complete workout
- y*outh booster,* a technique designed to rejuvenate you in an area where the aging process may be causing you to deteriorate
- *energy pack*, foods that are able to boost your energy levels
- *Rx response*, a particular medical treatment that requires the intervention of a physician

Each of these targeting categories is intended to provide a specific set of responses to particular health problems or concerns. For example:

Do you suffer from jet lag? There's a quick fix in Chapter 4 recommending special exercise strategies and other responses.

Do you frequently lack energy? There's a youth booster Energy Scale in Chapter 3 to get you back on track.

Do you want to increase your physical strength and endurance significantly—even though you are past age sixty-five? A stamina strategy in Chapter 8 says you can.

Is your creativity lagging, or your emotional mood flat? Check the pick-me-up in Chapter 5.

You may be wondering whether there is a scientific basis for this approach to enhancing youth.

The targeting strategies that I'll be teaching can be traced to the specialized and sometimes secret training techniques employed by world-class athletes. To maximize their performance, these elite athletes rely on specificity training principles, which are designed to strengthen particular muscle groups, increase stamina, improve skills, and enhance emotional and psychological preparation for high-level competition.

For example, if a professional tennis player wants to improve the power of his serve in demanding tournament situations, he might first identify the particular shoulder and arm muscle groups he uses in serving. Then, he would work to strengthen those muscles in the weight room with exercises that mimic the serving motion. Also, this tennis player would most likely devote part of his workout to exercises that improve muscle stamina related to serving.

In addition, he would probably reexamine his diet, sleep habits, and other health practices to be sure that those support systems were being marshaled wisely to maximize serving precision and power. Finally, he might even evaluate his psychological well-being because in most cases physical performance is directly linked to one's emotional and mental state.

Ironically, my first serious exposure to this sort of training occurred not here in the United States, but in the secret athletic testing and training labs of the former Soviet Union.

FROM RUSSIA WITH AN IDEA

While on a research trip to Russia about twenty years ago, I was surprised when one of the officials there offered to give me an inside look at one of their closely guarded Olympic testing facilities for rowers. The Soviet scientists had designed these human fitness labs to try to wring the absolute maximum performance out of the human body during top-level athletic competition.

I watched in fascination as they demonstrated how they hooked up transducers, devices that convert physical movements and responses into electrical impulses, to parts of a rower's body. While the rower pulled an oar, these transducers transmitted electrical signals from the athlete's muscles to machines that measured which tissues were doing the most work.

Using such methods, the Soviet researchers and trainers could determine precisely the parts of the body that were contributing the most to increase the speed of the rowing shell. With this information, they were in a position to develop specific exercises that would target and develop the most important muscle groups for rowing—and thus improve the athlete's performance.

Of course, my observations about the Russian methods wouldn't have surprised our own Olympic coaches. We always knew that, in addition to the well-publicized and dangerous anabolic steroid treatments, the Soviets and the East Germans were also using legitimate specificity or "target" training techniques.

But this firsthand view of how the approach worked planted the seed of another idea in my mind—an idea with implications that go far beyond the training of an athlete. It dawned on me that the very same specialized training that was working so well for elite Soviet athletes might also work for those of us who live life on a less competitive physical level. The scientific literature is full of studies showing how targeting can transform people's ability to function in their daily lives.

For example, a study of Japanese nurses found that targeting can reduce work-related fatigue. The study established a link between poor arm strength and cardiovascular fitness and fatigue at the end of a workday. The researchers concluded that excessive fatigue could be treated in this group through exercises designed to increase arm strength and overall stamina. (See M. Shimaoka, et al., "Relationship of task strain and physical strength to end-of-work fatigue among nurses at social welfare facilities," *Sangyo Eiseigaku Zasshi*, July 1995, pp. 227–33.)

Research also indicates that targeting can develop the physical, emotional, and spiritual strength needed to meet specific job demands. Medical researchers have determined that physicians who treat cancer patients must focus on meeting their own physical, psychosocial, and spiritual needs. Otherwise, they may find they lack the stamina and depth of insight necessary to help their patients deal effectively with symptoms of advanced cancer. (See P. Story, "Symptom control in advanced cancer," *Seminal Oncology*, Dec. 1994, pp. 748–53.)

Targeting can reduce soreness and muscle damage during and after demanding specialized work tasks. Military special forces personnel, who had to perform missions involving downhill maneuvers, reduced their muscle soreness and damage by changing their training to include bouts of downhill running. (See P. G. Law, et al., "Downhill running to enhance operational performance in mountain terrain," NHRC Publication 94-36, U.S. Navy.)

Various studies have also shown that taking relatively high doses of vitamin E, in the 800 to 1200 IU range, before unaccustomed vigorous physical activity can reduce such soreness. In other words—as we'll see in Chapter 7—the targeting strategy can include nutrition and nutritional supplements as well as exercise.

MORE THAN A MERE WORKOUT

Targeting, as I have designed it for the average person, is more than a garden-variety physical fitness workout. It is a system of comprehensive home treatments and programs combining fundamental principles of exercise, nutrition, and preventive medicine that are designed to deal with such conditions and complaints as:

- fatigue
- obesity
- flagging memory
- lower back pain
- muscle and joint aches, including the discomforts of arthritis
- the inability of certain children to perform well at sports
- emotional ills, including depression and anxiety
- menopause symptoms
- sexual dysfunction
- high-risk profiles for many serious health conditions—including cardiovascular disease, various cancers, and osteoporosis
- childhood difficulties with physical or emotional development
- the gradual deterioration of the abilities of aging parents to function physically or mentally

The first step in formulating a targeting strategy—which is the master key to recapturing the power of youth—is to analyze your situation before you act on any health complaint. In other words, you should identify as precisely as possible the complaint or problem you face. Then you'll be in a better position to take the second step, which involves sorting through the possible responses or "treatments," many of which will be described in the following pages. These can help minimize or even cure the problem.

The targeting treatments we'll explore in the following pages involve a variety of techniques, which I summarized a few pages back and which are often highlighted in the boxes throughout the text. These include stamina strategies, quick fixes, pick-me-ups, energy packs, and fluid factoring. Here are some more details.

Stamina Strategies

The stamina strategies are a particular approach to targeting that makes use of a unique interface between aerobics and strength work. This combination produces higher levels of staying power in daily activities than either aerobics or strength work can produce alone.

A stamina strategy typically involves eight to ten minutes of specialized exercises designed to produce specific kinds of endurance and staying power that may be required by certain unexpected physical demands, such as excessive lifting, stretching, or walking.

The exercises may include a wide variety of movements, including:

- regular and reverse biceps curls with a moderately heavy object (such as a dictionary or light chair)
- bent-leg sit-ups
- special lumbar (lower back) stretches and strengthening moves

Stamina strategies are characterized by low-intensity, high-repetition movements that may combine limited endurance conditioning and strength training. The objective is to build stamina, or staying power, in various muscles throughout the body while minimizing the risk of injury to the aging "boomer" body.

Some of the most advanced new exercise machinery today is based on this low-intensity, high-repetition concept. But in this book, we'll focus whenever possible on workouts that involve little or no special equipment.

There has long been strong support in scientific literature for the endurance-strength-stamina link. For example, programs that emphasize both strength and endurance training have consistently worked well over the years in military conditioning programs. Recently, the U.S. Navy designed one of these strength-endurance regimens, which was followed over a ten-week period by a group of thirty sedentary men. The researchers found that the participants experienced significant gains in their muscular strength and staying power. (See J. McCarthy, et al., "Combined strength and endurance training: functional and morphological adaptation to ten weeks of training," NHRC Publication 92-26, U.S. Navy.)

Some common challenges that can be treated effectively with stamina strategies include:

- aches and pains resulting from office work done under great pressure
- heavier-than-normal physical work, such as moving furniture, carrying heavy suitcases for relatively long distances in an airport, or even toting an unusually heavy load of groceries
- playing for lengthy sessions with active children
- extended housework or yard work
- walking, climbing stairs, or otherwise engaging in an activity for a longer-than-normal period

But stamina strategies are just one of many possibilities we'll be considering as part of the targeting techniques in the following pages. Another powerful tool in preventing and treating youth drain—and recapturing the vigor of youth—is what I call the quick fix.

Quick Fixes

These exercises involve four or five minutes of special movements designed to overcome specific, short-term physical and emotional complaints.

For example, you might use a quick fix to overcome discomfort from a stiff back, fatigued or cramped hands, or temporary "fuzzyheadedness," any of which might result from several hours of prolonged concentration or work.

Quick-fix targeting often involves remedial stretches or high-repetition, low-intensity calisthenics. Sometimes, the movements can be performed with hand weights (weighing two and a half to five pounds) or with objects such as a broom, light chair, book, or empty suitcase.

Pick-Me-Ups

Typically, these involve four to five minutes of light but continuous activity designed to provide a lift during those periods of the day when your energy begins to flag.

Eye-Openers

These comfortable, but highly potent movements—with static stretches followed by a relatively painless, slow-build stamina-and-strength routine—help the "night owl" become more of an "early bird," or morning person.

Stopgaps

Sometimes, you know you need exercise to be at your best, but your work or travel pressures simply don't allow time for a full work-out outdoors or in the gym. In these situations, you can derive significant benefits from the stopgap strategy, which requires anywhere from five to twenty minutes of strength and aerobic work (such as jogging in place). This limited workout can be performed in the privacy of your home, your hotel room, or even your office.

Energy Packs

There are also nutritional strategies that can be used in a targeting program. One of these, the energy pack, focuses on special foods and snacks that have the power to both conserve and regulate your energy reserves.

For instance, if you find yourself running out of energy in the middle of the afternoon—and you're fairly certain your problem is nutritional rather than a lack of exercise—it's extremely important to pick your snack foods wisely. One targeting approach that a number of my patients have found to be quite effective is to key their snacks to the *glycemic index* of foods.

Generally speaking, those foods that are low on the glycemic index (such as fruits like orange and grapefruit) contain sugars that feed into the bloodstream more slowly than foods high on the index (such as commercially baked cookies or finely ground breads). The effect of this difference is that low glycemic index foods tend to stave off hunger longer than foods with a high glycemic index. Consequently, you're more likely to stave off your hunger pangs until dinnertime if you snack on an orange or a grapefruit than if you turn to chocolate chip cookies. Just as important, choosing a low glycemic index snack will tend to keep your intake of calories much lower than will a high index snack. (See *Journal of Applied Physiology*, Oct. 1993; 75[4]: pp. 1477–85; *Journal of Applied Physiology*, Jan. 1998; 84[1]: pp. 53–9.)

Foods that are low on the glycemic index—and thus tend to "stick with you" longer and keep those hunger pangs at bay—include grapefruit, oranges, cereals with a high wheat bran content, and cantaloupe.

Those that are high on the glycemic index—and that tend to feed sugars into your system much more quickly, with the result that you get hungry sooner—include regular whole wheat bread, English muffins, baked potatoes, flaked cereals, watermelon, yogurt, and carrots. (As you can see, even quite healthy foods may not be the best snacks when you are trying to make it to the next meal without being overwhelmed by hunger.)

Energy Pack
The Power of Fruit Sugars to Promote Endurance

In a 1988 study done at Sapporo Medical College in Japan, twelve trained men were divided into two groups. One group was given 60 to 85 grams of fructose (fruit sugar) sixty minutes before exercise while the other received a sweet placebo that did not contain fructose. The men were then required to do aerobic exercise to the point of exhaustion.

The difference in exercise times achieved by each of the two groups was dramatic. The group that had consumed the fructose lasted an average of 145 minutes for their exercise session while the placebo group averaged only 132 minutes.

The researchers concluded that fructose ingestion is of benefit before prolonged exercise because, by keeping blood sugars at a relatively high level, it helps delay fatigue. (See *Medical Science, Sports and Exercise*, April 1988; 20[2]: pp. 105–9.)

In a related study reported in the *Journal of Applied Physiology* in 1983, researchers compared the effect of ingesting fructose (fruit sugar), and glucose (simple sugars such as those found in commercial candies and cookies). They found that fructose ingested before thirty minutes of submaximal exercise maintained stable blood glucose (blood sugar) and insulin concentrations—a result that may lead to sparing of muscle glycogen and greater endurance. (See Dec. 1983; 55[6]: pp. 1767–71.)

(Note: When your body draws upon internal sugar stores for energy, the blood sugars are the first to be used. Then the sugar stored in the muscles is tapped; and finally, your body begins to use body fat. You're least likely to be distracted by hunger pangs or other physical discomforts when your body is drawing upon the sugars in your bloodstream.)

Fluid Factoring

Do you typically run out of steam before the day is finished? Or do you lose concentration toward the end of the workday? Do you panic under deadline pressure? Do you experience any stress-related health problems, such as back pains or headaches?

If so, you may simply need to consume more fluids. Fluid factoring is nothing more than being careful to manage the intake of liquids into your system throughout the day.

Targeting can keep your daily intake of fluids and electrolytes (salts and other chemicals such as sodium, potassium, and chlorides) high enough to prevent mild dehydration, which can lower energy levels. Fluid management is also necessary for such benefits as effective throat lubrication when you need a strong speaking voice.

Energy Pack
Keep Drinking When It's Cold

Even if you don't feel as sweaty when you're outside during cold weather, don't be fooled! Most likely, you're perspiring as much as you do in hot weather. The main difference is that the cold, dry air causes your skin to stay cooler and your perspiration to evaporate more efficiently.

Also, if you fail to drink when the weather is cold, you may very well find your energy levels decreasing, and your ability to work efficiently declining.

In a study done with recreational alpine skiers, researchers at the University of Colorado at Colorado Springs tested losses of fluid in temperatures of 14 to 48 degrees Fahrenheit, at altitudes of 8,000 to 10,500 feet. Half the skiers had constant access to drinking water while the other half had access to drinking water only during lunch breaks.

In this study the skiers who were able to drink water regularly reported feeling significantly better. Also, the ones without water experienced a decline in blood plasma of almost 5 percent, while those with water lost 0.1 percent.

Various studies have demonstrated that a loss of blood plasma can cause a decline in stamina and endurance, and other physical problems. In another report, published in the *Penn State Sports Medicine Newsletter,* reviewers noted that when a 150-pound athlete loses 2 percent of his body weight (about three pounds) during heavy exercise, his physical and mental performance may decrease by as much as 20 percent. (See *The New York Times*, Dec. 16, 1997, p. B17.)

How do these targeting strategies work in the real world?

Here is how one woman, whom I'll call "Diane," used a special configuration of these techniques to overcome some common complaints related to fatigue and job stress.

DIANE'S DILEMMA AND THE TARGETING TREATMENT THAT CHANGED HER LIFE

Diane was on the upswing at her company. She had just received a sizable raise and was being considered for a senior vice president's slot. As a result, she was traveling more, working longer hours when she was in the office, and seeing her family less and less.

The work achievements were exhilarating and satisfying, but the pressures were beginning to get to her. Diane had noticed that she was becoming more irritable, both at home and at work. As well as she could determine, her problems seemed to begin first thing every morning and then to grow worse as the day wore on.

Working effectively in the morning had been a problem for her since her college years, but now the situation was worse than she could ever remember. The demands of being a mother to two teenage children, an understanding and responsive wife, and a top-notch performer at work had become overwhelming. The stress was beginning to take its toll on her physically.

She had been feeling increasingly fuzzy-headed and tired well into the mid-morning hours, when she needed to think clearly and be more productive. She was also experiencing more lower back pains, leg aches, and stiffness in her muscles and joints.

Diane knew several factors were contributing to her problem. These included too little sleep, a sense that she wasn't getting enough help on domestic duties from her husband and children, and an inability to handle the bad stress in her life adequately.

Also, she was aware that she had become almost totally sedentary. From what she had read and heard, she decided that becoming more physically fit might be the best first step in helping her reduce her stress and get better sleep. Then, she could turn to the issue of negotiating more help at home. So she embarked on a personal fitness program at a local gym during her lunch hour.

Diane's analysis of her situation was right on target: regular exercise could go a long way toward solving her energy problems. Unfortunately, however, she ran into difficulty at the outset because she began to skip many of the scheduled workouts.

"It's a matter of priorities," she explained. "By the time I do the whole thing at the gym, including dressing and showering, I use well over an hour. So what's the choice? After I meet a late deadline at work, should I choose to spend my remaining hour or so of the day with the family? Or should I go to the gym and work out?"

I can't argue with her personal priorities—obviously, putting your family at the top of the list is a good idea. But when she put her fitness program on hold, she found herself right back where she had started—with high stress levels, poor sleep, and no alternate strategy to help begin to relieve her complaints.

What was she to do?

The solution lay not in trying to make time for a workout that would seldom mesh with her busy life, but in targeting. Targeting would allow her to develop an exercise routine that would fit into her packed daily schedule and put her on the track to reducing her physical and mental fatigue.

With her sporadic strength and aerobic work at the gym, Diane had already established a minimal base of conditioning—the basic fitness foundation I describe in Chapter 2. In other words, even though she wasn't in tip-top shape, she had moved beyond being totally sedentary. As a result, she was in a position to engage in a targeting strategy that had the potential to overcome her problems.

The most important change Diane made was to begin every day with an eye-opener—a light, ten- to fifteen-minute exercise routine designed to help people who are sluggish in the morning jump-start their day. Diane was by nature a night owl. In the mornings, she was exceptionally slow to get moving. She preferred to ease into the day, with as little physical activity or other outside demands as possible.

No special equipment was required for Diane's eye-opener routine. She simply started out on her bedroom rug with five to ten minutes of special static stretching movements, which research has shown can provide a number of early-morning benefits. These include greater all-body circulation; wider ranges of physical motion; reduction of stiffness, aches, and cramps; and increased ease of movement. (See S. Bentley, "Exercise-induced muscle cramp—proposed mechanisms and management," *Sports Medicine*, June 1996; 21[6]: pp. 409–20.)

Most people also find that a few minutes of the right kind of stretching the first thing in the morning can minimize or eliminate stiffness and physical aches throughout the day. Just as important, such a routine helps clear the mind and prevents mental slowness in the early-morning hours.

Quick Fix
Proven Techniques for Overcoming Stiffness

In a 1996 New Zealand study, twenty-four healthy, fit subjects who were experiencing stiffness in their feet and limited range of motion in their ankles were all assigned to three separate programs, in this order:

First, they did stretching movements for their ankles and feet, including five thirty-second static stretches, with a thirty-second rest between each stretch. Second, they did a short aerobic exercise routine: running on a treadmill for ten minutes at 60 percent of their maximum age-predicted heart rate. Third, they engaged in a combined protocol, first running and then stretching.

The results showed that running was more effective than stretching for decreasing muscle stiffness. But to increase the range of motion of their ankles, both the combination running-stretching protocol and the stretching protocol alone were more effective than the running alone. The researchers concluded that both jogging and static stretching exercises are beneficial to active individuals who experience stiffness and limits on the range of motion of their joints.

(See the *British Journal of Sports Medicine*, Dec. 1966; 30[4]: pp. 313–7.)

Diane began her stretches with a variation on what is sometimes called the "Williams exercises." I call my eye-opener version of these movements the "sleepyhead stretches" because they are specially targeted to ease the transition from sleep to significant physical activity.

(For a detailed description of the sleepyhead stretches, see Chapter 2.)

With this preliminary stretching sequence completed, Diane sat up very carefully and began a series of other slow stretches. These included hamstring stretches, upper arm and shoulder stretches, static Achilles tendon stretches, groin stretches, and lunges. (For details on how to do these stretches, see Chapter 2.)

At this stage of her eye-opener routine, Diane found that she had made a successful physical and mental transition from her usual sleepyhead condition. Now, she was ready for more exercise action, which would really get her blood flowing and prepare her for an energy-packed day.

Diane had already conditioned her upper body fairly well in the gym with bench presses and other chest exercises that required weight equipment. Also, she had done a fair amount of abdominal work involving sit-ups, regular crunches (partial sit-ups that condition the upper abdominal muscles), and crunches done against weight resistance. So as part of her eye-opener routine, she was able to plug in two final, rather rigorous strength-and-stamina exercises.

First, she did a series of bent-leg sit-ups. These were easy for her to switch to because she was already on the floor after having done her stretches. After she had finished enough sit-ups to cause a reasonable degree of fatigue in her abdominal muscles, she turned over on her stomach and performed as many modified push-ups (push-ups performed with the knees planted on the floor) as she could manage without resting. Then she relaxed for about twenty seconds and did a second set of modified push-ups.

The fifteen minutes allotted for Diane's morning workout had now elapsed, and she was ready to shower, have breakfast with her family, and head to work. The total time required for the continuous, nonstop eye-opener routine—which was a variation on more sophisticated "circuit training" used by many well-conditioned athletes—was relatively modest and could easily be inserted into her packed daily schedule.

Yet after her first experience in using the targeting approach to solve her early-morning woes, Diane wasn't so sure the strategy would work. In fact, she sensed she was actually feeling more fatigued than she had felt on the previous morning, when she had followed her normal routine.

When Diane mentioned these concerns to a friend who was a professional fitness trainer, the expert offered these wise words of caution: don't expect a dramatic turnaround after one day, or even after one week of any type of exercise, including this relatively undemanding eye-opener routine. Plan on at least two weeks, and preferably longer, to make a successful transition.

As for me, I always suggest that people embarking on a new workout regimen allow four to six weeks to establish the new habit and give their bodies time to adjust. Remember, too, that when you shift to a morning workout and you're not by nature a "morning person," you'll also have to give your body's circadian rhythms, or biological time clock, some extra time to get into sync.

Fortunately for Diane, she stuck with the program. As a result, after about two weeks the physical fatigue, leg aches, back pains, mental fuzziness, and other discomforts disappeared. She found she was starting off the day with a much higher level of energy and none of the fatigue that had plagued her before she began the eye-opener strategy. Most important of all, she could now think more clearly from the moment she set foot in the office until the time that she arrived back home at night.

To multiply her benefits, Diane began to experiment with additional targeting techniques, including some short pick-me-up routines late in the afternoon, when fatigue tended to overtake her. These included short, four- to five-minute sequences of modified push-ups, sit-ups, and running in place.

Diane understood, by the way, that the eye-opener and pick-me-up treatments for her energy, stiffness, and sleeping problems were not a substitute for a more serious fitness program. Even when her work schedule was packed, she still did her best to include a minimum of twenty minutes of aerobic work (such as fast walking, swimming, cycling, or jogging) three to four days a week. Also, when her occupational demands lessened a couple of months later, she returned to a regular, twice-a-week strength-and-flexibility routine at the fitness club she had joined.

But when the pressure was on, the special targeting responses Diane had chosen—the eye-opener and pick-me-up routines—were an effective temporary measure to enable her to maintain those high energy levels that characterize the power of youth.

This fitness program was by no means the ultimate solution for all Diane's concerns. She was wise enough to understand that she also had to be forthright with her family in explaining that she needed more support around the house. Also, she began to explore other stress-reduction strategies, such as those discussed in Chapters 3, 4, and 5. But the targeted fitness program she had chosen provided an extremely valuable first step to help her recover the energy that had been drained away by work and family concerns.

With this introduction to the power of youth and some of the targeting treatments that are available to achieve that power, you have an idea about where we are headed in this book. But before we plunge into the specifics, consider the following overview, which will give you a better idea about how to access some of the practical strategies of targeting.

How to Get the Most Out of This Book

Regaining the Power of Youth at Any Age has been designed to provide readers in the pre-boomer, baby-boomer, and post-boomer generations—roughly from about ages thirty-one to seventy-five—with a potent but easy-to-use manual for recapturing their lost or declining youthful vigor. Also, readers with family members who are younger than thirty or older than seventy-five will find guidelines for encouraging better health and fitness among loved ones in those age-groups.

The emphasis throughout will be on natural, noninvasive self-treatment, such as special exercise responses, nutritional strategies, and the development of a variety of healthy habits that have been proven effective through various studies in preventive medicine. Also, when self-treatment isn't appropriate because of the need for medications or other physician-directed procedures, the emphasis will be on assisting your doctor in pinpointing or diagnosing your particular problem.

In the next chapter, you'll be introduced to the "trilogy of targeting," basic fitness and dietary techniques that apply to those at all age levels. Then, in Chapter 3, you'll assess your power of youth by evaluating yourself according to the Cooper Energy Scale.

In the final three chapters of Part 1, you'll delve more deeply into these issues:

- youth drain—those factors that can rob anyone, even those younger than thirty, of the power of youth
- the secrets of stamina at every age—the hidden sources of energy that most people overlook
- the paralysis of medical confusion—the tendency to become immobilized by the often contradictory blizzard of medical information coming to us through the mass media

Part 2 of the book focuses on certain special health concerns—and targeting solutions—for a variety of different age-groups. First, we'll deal with the adults from thirty to seventy-five years old—an age range dominated by the boomer generation, those who were born between 1946 and 1964. Then, we'll switch our health spotlight to two other age-groups with special health concerns—those age seventy-six and above and those who are younger than thirty.

An emphasis in Part 2 will be on how boomers, who are likely to have some say in the health management of both the youngest and the oldest groups, can spot problems and communicate appropriate advice effectively. Also, we'll explore how you can collaborate with your doctor when medications or physician-initiated procedures are required to complete a targeting solution.

Major themes and features throughout these pages will include:

- common health complaints and conditions—and suggested treatments—that readers in particular age categories can expect to encounter
- specific, programmatic advice in the form of targeting strategies, which will focus on exercise and nutritional responses to particular health concerns. Many of these ideas and recommendations will appear in highlighted "boxes," such as those included in this first chapter
- the latest scientific findings on aging—and how you can make the best use of them
- a comprehensive plan to overcome one of the most common fears known to modern men and women—the fear of aging and old people, or *gerontophobia*, as it is sometimes called

Now, let's begin our exploration with a consideration of the three basic tools of targeting, which should be understood and employed by men and women of every age—striking, strengthening, and stretching. After you learn how to use these strategies, you'll be well on your way to regaining the power of youth, regardless of how old you are.

2
· · · · · · · · · · · · ·

Strike, Strengthen, and Stretch: The Basic Targeting Trilogy

Regardless of your age, if you hope to infuse your life with the power of youth, you must learn to apply the three *S*'s of targeting—striking, strengthening, and stretching.

First of all, following a strike-strengthen-stretch program will provide you with the basic level of fitness you need to age slowly and maintain maximum physical functioning. Second, this basic trilogy includes most of the fitness responses or "treatments" that will help you deal with many physical and emotional concerns and complaints.

As I use the three terms here, each requires some further explanation. As we proceed, we'll examine how the strike-strengthen-stretch trilogy represents a coordinated response to such challenges as:

- the loss of bone mass during aging—which can be countered with "striking" (impact) activity
- the loss of muscle mass—which can be overcome through an age-adjusted "Aerobic-Strength Axis"

- the decline of cardiovascular power—which can be slowed through endurance conditioning
- the need to base an effective, long-term fitness program on a cross-training concept
- the importance of drawing up a "targeting guide" to deal with your specific health concerns and problems

Now, let's explore the meaning of the first component of the targeting trilogy—striking.

PART ONE: STRIKE

By *striking*, I mean exercise with impact. Impact occurs in many activities, such as when:

- a jogger's foot strikes the ground
- a tennis player's racket strikes the ball
- an aerobic dancer jumps
- a volleyball player returns a serve
- a boxer slugs a punching bag

Why is striking so important?

One major reason is that striking is essential to effective bone building and bone mass maintenance. Thinning of the bones makes you more vulnerable to injuries and may eventually lead to osteoporosis, the disease of aging characterized by excessive loss of bone density.

Another reason striking exercise is important is that it often promotes endurance or aerobic training. Although aging inevitably results in a loss of cardiovascular power, you can take steps to slow or stop this deterioration—and impact often provides the best answer.

Here are some of the details on these two benefits of striking.

Building Youthful Bones Through Striking

Bone mass declines at an estimated annual rate of 0.3 to 0.5 percent after about age thirty to forty, and that loss accelerates to 2 to 3 percent for women during an eight- to ten-year period after they go through menopause.

During their entire lives, women lose about 35 percent of their cortical bone mass (such as the long bones of the arms and legs) and 50 percent of the trabecular bone mass (such as the vertebrae). Men will lose almost a quarter of their cortical bone mass and about one-third of their trabecular bone.

How can this loss of bone be slowed?

First of all, it's absolutely essential to get involved in striking types of exercise as early as you can. The longer you wait—and the older you become—the more bone density you will lose.

It is well known that you can reduce the loss of bone mass by increasing your calcium intake, going on hormone replacement therapy (HRT) if you are a woman who has entered menopause, or avoiding such bone-damaging substances as smoking and alcohol.

But perhaps the most important and fundamental response—one that works well by itself and even better when combined with good nutrition and other healthy habits and medical treatments—is impact exercise.

Although this type of exercise has sometimes been referred to as *weight-bearing* exercise, that term isn't quite precise. It's actually the impact that produces the benefit to the body's bone mass. Weight merely adds to the impact experienced during certain types of exercise.

Consider the conclusions of a 1996 German study that compared the bone mass of three groups of athletes: weight lifters, boxers, and bicycle racers.

When compared with a group of controls (nonathletes), the weight lifters showed a 23 percent increase in bone density in the neck of the femur bone ("Ward's triangle"), which is situated near the hip. The boxers had an increase of 17 percent in the lower (lumbar) spine, 9 percent in the hip, and 7 percent in the neck of the femur.

But the bicycle racers, when compared with the controls, actually showed a bone mineral *decrease* of 10 percent in the lumbar spine, 14 percent in the hip, and 17 percent in the neck of the femur. (See *Z Orthop Ihre Grenzgeb*, Jan. 1996; 134[1]: pp. 1–6.)

Why the differences among these athletes? There are several possible explanations. First of all, the increase in bone density in the weight lifters and boxers appears to confirm the effects of striking-type exercise. In other words, as the boxers move and dance about, their spines and hips undergo weight-bearing impact, which helps build up bones. The same is true for competitive weight lifters, who experience impact when they lift maximum amounts of weight.

The bicycle riders, in contrast, experience no significant impact as they pedal; so their sport, as great as it is for building cardiovascular endurance, does little for their bone development. Also, because they are endurance athletes, the cyclists tend to have an extremely low amount of body fat. Consequently, they tend to weigh less than the average nonathletic controls—a condition that places less bone-building stress on their skeletal structures as they pursue their ordinary daily activities.

Another study conducted in 1997 at the University of North Carolina focused on the effect of six months of heavy weight lifting on premenopausal women forty to fifty years old. The researchers found that the women assigned to the weight-lifting program, which was designed to place strain on the spine and hips, experienced a 1.03 percent increase in the bone density of their lumbar spine. In contrast, a control group that didn't exercise suffered a 0.36 percent decline in lumbar bone density.

The study concluded that even a short-term weight-training program can maintain or even improve bone mineral density in parts of the body that are exposed to the most mechanical pressure. (See *Journal of Sports Medicine and Physical Fitness,* Dec. 1997; 37[4]: pp. 246–51.)

In a 1991 Duke University study, researchers explored the effect of up to fourteen months of aerobic exercise on bone density in older adults. The project involved 101 healthy men and women over age sixty (with a mean age of sixty-seven) who either engaged in an exercise program (stretching, cycling, and walking three times per week for sixty minutes) or were involved in nonaerobic programs.

The researchers found that the exercise training produced a 10 to

32

15 percent increase in cardiovascular aerobic power after four months and a 1 to 6 percent further improvement with additional training. Also, the aerobic fitness program produced significant bone density increases in the men, but not in the women. (See *Journal of the American Geriatric Society*, Nov. 1991; 39[11]: pp. 1065–70.)

In fact, a number of studies have revealed that men—particularly older men—tend to respond to lower-impact exercise with increases in their bone density while women do not. With women—particularly older women—some sort of mechanical impact, such as jumping, hitting a ball, or running, usually seems to be required for bone building.

The reasons for this gender difference in the bone-building effects of lower-impact exercise aren't clear. One possible explanation is that because men tend to have more lean body mass, they are able to put more explosive force on their skeletal structure when they exercise. The impact stimulates the reproduction of bone cells, which increase the buildup of bone density.

Additionally, in a 1996 Swedish study of female soccer players, researchers found that the athletic women had significantly higher bone mineral density in certain key areas of their skeletal structure than did a group of nonactive female controls. (See *Calcified Tissue International*, Dec. 1996; 59[6]: pp. 438–42.)

The investigators determined that there was a site-specific skeletal response to "loading" imposed by running and kicking motions. In particular, the soccer players had significantly higher bone mineral density in these sites: lumbar (lower) spine, 10.7 percent; femoral (upper thigh bone) neck, 13.7 percent; soft tissue at the top of the femur, 19.6 percent; and tibia (shinbone), 12 percent.

Interestingly, however, the researchers determined that muscle strength in the thigh was not related to bone mass in the female soccer players. In other words, the key fact for bone building was mechanical impact, not muscle strength.

A 1997 Australian study of mature female athletes, ages forty-two to fifty, found that women who participate regularly in their premenopausal years in high-impact physical activity tend to have higher bone density than nonathletic women. (See *Medical Science, Sports and Exercise*, March 1997; 29[3]: pp. 291–6.)

In this investigation, one group of women was involved in high-impact sports (volleyball or basketball); a second group participated in moderate-impact sports (running and field hockey); a third was engaged in a nonimpact sport (swimming); and a fourth group was a nonathletic control group.

The high- and moderate-impact groups had significantly higher whole-body bone mineral density than the controls. Also, both impact groups had greater leg bone mineral density than the swimmers.

A 1996 study conducted at the Mayo Clinic, Rochester, Minnesota, focused on the effect of exercise on bone mineral density of the spine in premenopausal women ages thirty to forty. (See *Bone*, Sept. 1996; 19[3]: pp. 233–44.)

Women in an exercise group performed supervised, nonstrenuous weight-lifting exercises twice a week. Also, they exercised twice a week on their own. A control group didn't exercise.

The researchers determined that the exercise increased muscle strength but had no significant effect on the bone mineral density at the spine, hip, or middle of the forearm.

This study confirms other reports that while low-impact strength training may increase muscle strength in women, there is little or no direct effect on bone building.

As you've undoubtedly noticed, there's an apparent inconsistency between the effect that strength training has on a man's bones and the effect that it has on a woman's bones. In short, some studies have shown that such strength workouts result in higher bone density for men but not for women. What's going on here?

In a 1996 study that dealt directly with this issue in young women, twenty females averaging about twenty years of age participated in a weight-training program involving upper- and lower-body exercises twice per week for twenty weeks.

The researchers from McMaster University in Hamilton, Ontario, determined that a resistance training program did effectively increase strength and lean tissue in the young women. For example, they experienced an increase in strength in the arm curl (73 percent), bench press (33 percent), and leg press (23 percent).

But the female exercisers did not have an increase in their bone mineral content or density over the training period. (See *Canadian Journal of Physiology and Pharmacology*, Oct. 1996; 74[1]: pp. 1180–5.)

This issue of bone building in women is complicated somewhat by an observation, made by some researchers, that women's muscle strength can be a predictor of their bone mineral density. That is, if a woman is relatively strong, with a high proportion of lean muscle mass, it is more likely, from a statistical viewpoint, that she'll have stronger bones than a weaker woman.

A probable reason for this result is the indirect effect that becoming stronger can have on anyone's bones, male or female. In other words, the strong woman can exert more mechanical pressure on her bones than a weaker woman. So even though strength training in itself may not increase bone density in women as much as in men, women who develop more powerful muscles from such training are more likely to be able to exert more striking impact during their workouts. For that matter, they can apply more mechanical force while pursuing their ordinary daily activities, such as participating in recreational sports or doing work around the house. Consequently, they are able to put more pressure on their skeletal structure and are thus more likely to increase their bone mass.

To sum up, here are the highlights of these various findings on the effects of striking:

- Striking, or impact-type exercise, tends to build up bone density in both men and women in skeletal sites that are subjected to mechanical pressure.
- Men's bones respond more to lower-impact endurance exercise, including strength work, than do women's—possibly because of the ability of more muscular males to exert additional pressure on their bones during a lower-impact workout.
- In both men and women, stronger muscles are predictors of

higher bone density—and may also have an indirect effect on building bone mass.

Men and women of all ages should include striking-type exercise in their program to maximize their bone mass now and to retard the inevitable loss of bone mass during aging. Good striking exercises for both men and women include jogging, tennis, volleyball, aerobic dance, canoeing, rope skipping—basically any type of activity that involves impact.

Men may also derive significant bone-building benefits from lower-impact strength training, such as lower-intensity weight lifting involving high repetitions with light weights. Women should engage in this type of workout as well to build up their muscles. But to gain the additional benefit of bone building from strength work, they will probably have to rely on high-intensity weight training (with relatively heavy weights and low repetitions) or on aerobic exercises that also build muscles and bones.

For both men and women, it's best to get the three-pronged combination effect of 1) endurance training, 2) strength training, and 3) bone building. To achieve this end, endurance exercise, with both striking (impact) and strength-building components, is the ideal. Jogging, canoeing, and tennis all fit this category.

Please note this word of caution: higher-impact exercise does carry a greater risk of injury than a lower-impact workout. So if you plan to embark on a striking-oriented program, be sure also to focus on strength training that will help you build up supporting muscles, ligaments, and other tissues.

Also, monitor your body's danger signals by "listening" to your body. If you notice muscle, skeletal, ligament, or joint pains that last more than two or three days, take a break from the impact exercise. To maintain your aerobic power and get some added strength work during this break, substitute a low-impact activity, such as swimming. If the pain or discomfort continues, see a qualified physician.

Be aware that aerobic exercise triggers the release of endorphins, morphine-like neurotransmitters that can mask pain from an injury for two to four hours after a workout. So before you can begin to evaluate the nature of an injury, you should wait for the endorphin effect to wear off.

Now, let's move on to the next component of our targeting trilogy—strengthening—which, as we've already discussed, is closely related to the bone-building and endurance issues.

PART TWO: STRENGTHEN

This second leg in the basic targeting trilogy involves increasing the strength and power of the various muscle groups throughout your body.

As we've already seen, building bone mass is an essential part of maintaining the vigor of youth. If your bones can't support your body—and especially if they break easily—your ability to function will be greatly impaired. But building muscle is just as important: lean body mass provides us with the power and strength we need to continue to move, lift, and maneuver in our older years as effectively as we did when we were in our teens or twenties.

Still, what builds our bones doesn't necessarily build all the muscles we need. Also, strength work should always be combined with aerobic or endurance conditioning. This balance of aerobic power and muscular strength—through what I call the Aerobic-Strength Axis—is central to any understanding of how strength training operates in any power of youth program.

THE AEROBIC-STRENGTH AXIS

To design a personal fitness program that will enable you to maintain the highest levels of youthful vigor and energy, it's absolutely necessary to be guided by the Aerobic-Strength Axis, which can be stated this way: include both aerobic (endurance) and strength training in your weekly workout program. When you are younger, weight your regimen in favor of aerobic training. As you grow older, shift the emphasis toward strength training.

The reason that this principle is so important is that your muscle mass and strength will inevitably decline as you grow older. At first, up to about age fifty, you will lose only about 4 percent of your strength and muscle mass per decade. But after that, the loss increases to about 10 percent per decade.

By age sixty, according to Dr. Herbert Haupt, a St. Louis orthopedic surgeon who has done research in this area, the average man will have lost about one-third of his muscle mass—unless he takes countermeasures such as those I'm suggesting in this book. (See *Barron's*, June 8, 1998, p. H6.)

But the muscles aren't the only part of your body that begins to deteriorate with age. Another effect of aging is the steady erosion of *oxygen uptake*, the ability of the lungs, heart, and cardiovascular system to process oxygen during endurance exercise. The higher your oxygen uptake, the more aerobic power and overall stamina you have—and that's an essential goal for anyone who wants to recover the power of youth.

Here are some findings about what happens to your endurance as you grow older—and why these changes take place:

A variety of studies have established that maximal aerobic capacity declines regularly with age for both aerobically fit and unfit men and women. According to a 1998 study at the Baltimore Veterans Affairs Medical Center, Baltimore, all men lose about 9 percent of their aerobic power per decade from about age forty-five to age eighty. (See *Journal of Applied Physiology*, June 1998; 84[6]: pp. 2163–70.)

Women face a similar decline. A 1997 study at the Department of Kinesiology, University of Colorado, found that both trained and untrained women, ages twenty to seventy-five, lost about 9 to 10 percent of their aerobic power per decade. (See *Journal of Applied Physiology*, July 1997; 83[1]: pp. 160–5.)

There is solid evidence, however, that endurance training can make a difference. In the first place, even though a number of studies indicate that both fit and unfit men and women lose their endurance at the same rate, fit people start off at a higher level. As a result, in absolute terms, they retain more aerobic power than their unfit counterparts over the years.

Also, there is evidence that highly trained endurance athletes can head off the loss of aerobic power as they age more effectively than those who are less fit. A 1990 study at the Washington University School of Medicine, St. Louis, published in the *Journal of Applied Physiology* (May 1990; 68[5]: pp. 2195–9), focused on a group of fifteen highly trained endurance athletes, averaging about sixty-two years of age. These athletes, who were followed for about eight years, lost aerobic power at a calculated rate of only 5.5 percent per decade. In contrast, a control group of fourteen sedentary people lost aerobic power at a rate of about 12 percent per decade.

In a similar vein, the 1996 report of a twenty-two-year study at the Human Performance Laboratory at Ball State University in Muncie, Indiana, showed that the aerobic capacity of highly trained middle-aged men declined by only 5 to 7 percent per decade.

It may be possible to use endurance training to slow the loss of endurance capacity even more dramatically. In a February 1987 report in the *Journal of Applied Physiology* (Vol. 62, No. 2, pp. 725–31), researchers followed over a ten-year period a group of track athletes who remained highly competitive. The aerobic capacity of the athletes, who ranged in age from fifty to eighty-two, remained unchanged during the entire ten-year period.

As for me, I can calculate rather precisely from the decline in my performance on treadmill stress tests, which measure cardiovascular and aerobic capacity, that my aerobic power has dropped a total of about 10 percent over a twenty-seven-year period. That amounts to a loss of approximately 3 to 4 percent per decade.

Another interesting finding that has emerged from a number of these studies is a link between the loss of endurance during aging and an increase in body fat. As a general rule for both men and women, when the percent of body fat goes up, the aerobic power goes down. (See companion studies of men, ages twenty-five to seventy, and women, ages twenty to sixty-four, in *Medical Science, Sports and*

Exercise, Jan. 1995; 27[1]: p. 113–20; and July 1996, 28[7]: pp. 884–91.)

The location of fat also seems to be an issue in the loss of endurance during aging. In a 1995 Baltimore study, increasing waist circumference with age in both men and women was strongly associated with declines in leisure time physical activity and peak endurance capacity. (See *Archives of Internal Medicine*, Dec. 11, 1995; 155[22]: pp. 2443–8.) In other words, aging plus less exercise equals more body fat (especially around the waist) and lower levels of endurance.

Clearly, both strength and aerobic training can make a huge difference in helping you hold off the physical deterioration of aging and regain much of the energy and youthfulness you enjoyed when you were much younger. But it won't do just to set up an aerobic-and-strength program for a thirty year old and expect it to work properly for someone who is forty, fifty, or sixty. Our endurance and muscle needs are quite different at different ages, and any fitness program must be designed to accommodate these variations. For your fitness program to work properly, it will be necessary to achieve just the right balance for your age between aerobic and strength work.

After studying the available scientific literature and evaluating my own experience with endurance and strength training over more than three decades, I've arrived at some conclusions about how strength training and endurance exercise should be adjusted for different age-groups. Here are the percentages of aerobic versus strength work that I suggest for different age ranges. These percentages should be understood in terms of time spent working out during a given week.

- age forty and younger: 80 percent aerobic, 20 percent strength
- ages forty-one to fifty: 70 percent aerobic, 30 percent strength
- ages fifty-one to sixty: 60 percent aerobic, 40 percent strength
- ages sixty-one and older: 55 percent aerobic, 45 percent strength

So if your age recommendation involves 80 percent aerobic and 20 percent strength work, that would mean that with a total of 2.5 hours

lished in the *Journal of the American Medical Association* (Nov. 3, 1989, pp. 2395–401). Furthermore, the more fit you are, the greater your ability to function effectively and youthfully as you grow older.

The basic rule of thumb for minimal aerobic or endurance exercise, which scientific research and government recommendations confirm, is that you should do twenty to thirty minutes of aerobic activity three to four days a week.

There is some disagreement about whether the twenty to thirty minutes should be done all at once or if it may be done in segments of about ten minutes each. I am convinced that it's best to do this endurance activity continuously during each exercise session. In other words, if you've chosen to walk briskly for thirty minutes, four times a week, you should perform each of your walking sessions in one uninterrupted half hour.

The best endurance activities for most people tend to be walking, jogging, swimming, cycling, aerobic dance, and walking or jogging on a treadmill. To get adequate benefits, you may choose to keep things as simple as possible, without reference to specific regimens for particular sports or activities. If your ambitions are fairly modest, you could just go out and take a vigorous walk for twenty or thirty minutes three to four days per week. That will provide you with a basic minimum level of health benefits and a significant chance for a longer life.

But for additional benefits and a greater potential to increase personal energy, you should do more. For more details, see the graduated programs involving a variety of different activities that are described in my books *Faith-Based Fitness* (Chapter 7; Thomas Nelson Publishers, 1995) and *Antioxidant Revolution* (Chapter 4; Thomas Nelson Publishers, 1994).

The Strength Side of the Axis

As you grow older, the need to do strength training becomes increasingly important to help you retard the loss of muscle and bone mass. But I strongly advocate getting started in this area when you are young. By starting young, you'll develop a solid set of habits—and muscles—to build upon as you age.

There are many ways to build your muscle strength, and I've included many detailed programs in *Faith-Based Fitness* (Chapter 8) and *Antioxidant Revolution* (Chapter 5). But getting started and building a base of muscle strength is a relatively simple matter that doesn't require a comprehensive, complicated program.

If you don't have access to a gym, with trainers and various types of machines, here's an easy start-up strength program that I suggest:

Bent-leg sit-ups or crunches. Do as many as you can until you become comfortably tired. Then rest about one minute and do as many more as you can. Try adding extra repetitions about every three sessions.

Push-ups. You can do modified push-ups (with knees on the floor) or regular push-ups (with back and legs straight, knees off the floor when you push your body up off the floor with your hands). Again, do as many as you can, rest about a minute, and then "max out" one more time. As with the sit-ups, after about three sessions, add extra repetitions.

Curls. Do arm curls with light dumbbells. The weights should be light enough to allow you to do at least eight repetitions without stopping, but heavy enough so that you can't easily exceed ten repetitions. Add repetitions over several sessions until you reach twelve to fifteen repetitions. Then add an extra "set" (another group of consecutive repetitions, done after a one-minute rest). When you are able to do two or three sets of twelve to fifteen repetitions, begin again with a slightly heavier set of weights.

Lunges. To execute lunges, begin by standing up straight, with arms spread out from your sides for balance. Let your body fall forward, and "catch" yourself by thrusting your left foot and leg out in front of your body. Let your body fall as far forward as possible, but don't allow your left knee to be bent beyond a ninety-degree angle. Do eight to ten repetitions with the left leg, and then repeat with the right leg.

Again, these exercises are about as simple and basic as you can get.

But you'll be amazed at how your strength increases after you've followed this routine for only a month or so.

When you have established a basic foundation of strength by doing these exercises for a couple of months, you may want to crank the challenge up a notch or two. To this end, you might select a more advanced program from one of my other books, which I've referred to in the previous discussion. Or you might join a gym and take advantage of the wide variety of exercise apparatuses now available. In any event, developing a more extensive strength program is almost always necessary as you grow older.

Finally, keep in mind the importance of the first element in the targeting trilogy, striking or impact-oriented exercise. As you've seen, you can select a striking-type exercise that can also provide the benefits of aerobic and strength training. Or perhaps even better, you can alternate high-impact exercise with medium- or low-impact exercise, such as walking, cycling, or swimming.

We'll go into more detail on this idea when we discuss the *cross-training concept*. But first, let's take a close look at the third component in the trilogy—stretching.

PART THREE: STRETCH

One of the most overlooked and misunderstood elements in a sound physical fitness program is the development of flexibility, the third and final component of the targeting trilogy.

One reason for this mistake is that relatively few definitive studies have been done on the benefits of stretching exercises, which enhance flexibility. Fitness researchers and trainers are constantly wrestling with such questions as these:

- *Question:* Is it necessary to do flexibility exercises as part of a warm-up program, prior to endurance work such as running or cycling?
  Answer: No. Other types of warm-ups, which begin to raise the heart rate and prepare the various muscle groups, can work just

as well. (For an example, see the box in Chapter 1 on how jogging, especially slow jogging, can be as effective as static stretching in warming up for a sports event.)

- *Question:* Does stretching help prevent injuries incurred during
  strength or aerobic training?
  Answer: The jury is still out on this issue, but my opinion is that
  stretching does help protect you against ligament and muscle
  injuries.
- *Question:* Will stretching help relieve aches and pains and energize me when I'm feeling fatigued?
  Answer: Yes, absolutely.
- *Question:* Will becoming more flexible help me recover a youthful range of motion and other signs of the power of youth
  throughout my body?
  Answer: Yes, absolutely.

So what exactly do we know about stretching and flexibility—and
how can we put this knowledge to some practical use?

First of all, let me say a word about the relationship between
flexibility and sports injury and performance. There is some scientific evidence to suggest that an active warm-up, including
stretching exercises, may be protective against most strain injuries.
On the other hand, being less flexible may improve running speed
and generation of force and power in certain types of athletic activities. (See *Sports Medicine*, Nov. 1997; 25[5]: pp. 289–99.)

Some experts also suggest that stretching and proper warm-up may
help protect the most commonly injured muscles—the hamstring (the
back of the thigh), the rectus femoris (from the hipbone over the front
of the thigh to the knee), the gastrocnemius (the back of the lower
leg), and the adductor longus (from the pubic bone down through the
inner thigh). (See the *American Journal of Sports Medicine*, 1996;
24[6 Suppl]: pp. S2–S8.)

In fact, a convincing body of scientific evidence supports the
validity of stretching as an essential component of any fitness routine. Here are some of the findings:

A 1994 study published in *Nursing Research* (July 1994; 43[4]: pp. 207–11) focused on a group of twenty elderly subjects who participated in eight weeks of low-intensity exercise, including stretching and strengthening movements. Another twenty-seven participants, who did no special exercises, functioned as a control group for comparison purposes.

The researchers found that the stretching group experienced significantly more flexibility of the ankles and knees, and they also improved their balance by 22 percent.

Tension-type headaches were relieved with a combination treatment of stretching the cervical (neck) spine muscles, massage, isotonic home exercises (exercises done against a constant level of resistance, such as doing sit-ups or lifting dumbbells), and education in use of better posture at home and work. (See *Headache*, March 1996; 36[3]: pp. 149–53.)

Stretching, combined with strengthening and aerobic conditioning exercises, can help reduce symptoms and in some cases relieve pain in patients with rheumatoid arthritis (inflammation of the joints linked to immune system problems) and osteoarthritis (wear-and-tear arthritis that occurs with overuse of the joints during aging). (See *Baillieres Clinical Rheumatology*, Feb. 1994; 8[1]: pp. 161–89.)

Youth Booster
Can Stretching Reverse Loss of Flexibility Due to Aging?

Stretching can help aging bodies regain some of their flexibility, according to a University of Wisconsin report in the *Archives of Physical and Medical Rehabilitation* (April 1988; 69[4]: pp. 268–72).

The investigators noted that decreased range of motion due to a lack of use can limit an older adult's ability to perform daily activities. They evaluated the flexibility of five joints in forty-six women ages sixty-five to eighty-nine before and after a twenty-five-week exercise program. The participants were divided into three groups: 1) controls who did no exercise; 2) women who exercised with light weights; and 3) women who exercised with no weights.

The results showed that both groups who exercised gained significantly greater range of motion in their ankles, shoulders, and neck rotation. The only difference between the two exercise treatments was that the group without weights gained significantly more range of motion in their shoulders than those who used light weights.

The researchers speculated that the reason for this difference might have been that the weights limited the movements of the participants' shoulders during the exercise.

They concluded that because other studies have suggested an age-related loss of flexibility in the shoulder, stretching exercises for the shoulder may be capable of reversing the loss of flexibility due to disuse.

This study clearly supports the point that stretching exercises are an essential component in any program that is intended to recover or maintain the functionality and physical capacity of youth.

So how should you stretch? Several types of stretching have been recommended and tried over the years. These include static stretching (holding a stretched-out position for twenty to thirty seconds); ballistic stretching (bouncing rather rapidly back and forth from a relaxed to a stretched position—an approach I do not recommend because of the increased danger of injury); and most recently the *dynamic range of motion* (DROM) stretch.

This last technique involves moving the body part to be stretched slowly through a full range of motion. For example, for a DROM right hamstring stretch, follow this procedure:

Lie on your back. Then raise your right leg off the floor, with your thigh at a right angle to your hip and the lower part of your leg bent at a ninety-degree angle. Slowly extend the lower part of your right leg so that your entire leg is extended at a right angle to your hip.

Hold this position, which places the greatest stretching pressure on the hamstring, for about five seconds. Finally, return the lower part of the right leg to the starting position. Repeat six times with the right leg, and then follow the same procedure six times with the left leg.

This DROM exercise for the hamstring was compared to regular static stretching in a 1998 study conducted at the University of Central Arkansas involving fifty-eight subjects twenty-one to forty-one years old. The researchers had the DROM stretchers do their movements five days a week. A second group did thirty-second static stretches with each leg five times a week. And a group of controls didn't stretch at all.

After six weeks of training, the investigators tested the flexibility of the subjects and found that even though both the static and DROM techniques improved flexibility, the static approach was superior. In fact, the static approach increased the range of motion by more than two times that of the DROM method. (See *Journal of Orthopedic Sports and Physical Therapy*, April 1998; 27[4]: pp. 295–300.)

In line with these findings, my own preference is for the static stretches.

What sort of program should you establish for yourself?

Here's a simple program that can provide the foundation for your basic workout routine. I suggest that you do these in the morning, just after you arise from bed, perhaps as an eye-opener to get started in the morning.

Sleepyhead Stretches

I introduced these stretches in Diane's example in Chapter 1. These are the best exercises I have encountered to prevent problems of the lower back. The sleepyhead stretches involve a sequence of four separate, highly effective—but, I might also add, very undemanding—movements. I've found that night owls are much more likely to get started with morning exercises if their first physical efforts in the morning are extremely easy.

In this case, the movements are as much like lying in bed as you can possibly make them! Yet they are among the very best exercises to prevent lower back problems.

Since I've developed the habit of doing a similar version of these stretches for the past decade or so, my stress-related lower back complaints have completely disappeared. Also, like Diane, I typically do them at the beginning of the day. They act as a highly effective targeting treatment to relax and energize me for a packed day of work.

If you need to get off the starting blocks in the morning, the sleepyhead stretch movements are made to order.

First, just after you arise in the morning, lie flat on your back on the floor. Close your eyes, relax for a few moments, and let the tension and stiffness seep out of your spine and muscles.

Then, wrapping both hands around your right knee, pull your right knee toward your chest until you feel steady but comfortable tension through your buttocks and lower back. Holding your knee as close to your chest as you can manage for ten to fifteen seconds, rock gently to your right and left to enhance the impact of the stretching on your spine. As you do this, you can feel the vertebrae in your spine "pop" and then relax further as though you are receiving a massage.

Next, lower your right leg back to a flat position on the floor, raise your left knee toward your chest, and perform similar stretching movements in this position for ten to fifteen seconds. End this second phase of your sleepyhead stretch routine by lowering your left leg to the floor.

Begin the third phase by pulling both knees toward your chest and holding them there for ten to fifteen seconds, rocking gently back and forth to maximize the stretching action on your spine, lower back, buttocks, and various muscle groups in your arms, shoulders, back, and legs. Finally, complete your introductory sleepyhead stretch while still on your back by shifting your legs up into a bent-leg position, with feet flat on the floor. Then press the small of your back against the floor, so that your entire spine is touching the ground, and hold this position for ten to fifteen seconds.

Static Achilles Tendon Stretches

To do these stretches, stand approximately four feet from a wall or other sturdy vertical structure. Move your left foot about halfway toward the wall, so that you seem to be taking a step forward. Both sets of toes should be pointing toward the wall.

Place both palms against the wall, with fingers pointed toward the ceiling.

Lean forward so that most of your weight bears down on your left foot and your hands. You should feel increasing tension on the back of your lower right leg and ankle, including the Achilles tendon. Hold this position for fifteen to twenty seconds.

Shift positions and perform the same stretch with your left leg back and your right leg forward.

Static Hamstring Stretches

Sit on the floor with legs straight out in front of you in a V. Your left foot should be positioned at a ninety-degree angle to the floor, with the toes pointing straight toward the ceiling. Now, bend your right leg and place your right foot flat against the side of your left knee.

Remaining in this position, you'll now perform several slow, static stretches. To maximize the benefits, hold each stretch for about fifteen seconds before going on to the next one.

First, extend both hands as far as you can toward your left ankle. Hold for fifteen to twenty seconds. Next, reach as far toward your left toes as you can with your left hand. Hold for fifteen to twenty seconds. Finally, reach as far as you can toward the toes with your right hand—and simultaneously twist your body slowly to the left and turn your head as far as you can manage in that direction, so that you are actually looking back to the rear.

Shift position and perform the same slow movements with your right leg extended forward.

Upper Arm and Shoulder Stretches

Begin in a sitting position on the floor, with your right arm extended above your head. Now, bend your right arm at the elbow and move your right hand as far down your back as you can, as if you are scratching your back.

To increase the tension on the back of your right arm and right shoulder, grasp your bent right elbow with your left hand and pull down and to the side, so that your right hand extends slightly farther down your back.

Finally, shift position and perform the same movements on the other side, so that your left hand is doing the back-scratching.

Groin Stretches

To do these, sit on the floor with your knees bent and the soles of your feet against each other. Holding both sets of toes together with your hands, pull your heels up as close to your groin as you can manage. At the same time, push down on the inside of your knees with your elbows. You should feel tension throughout your groin and inner thighs. Hold this position for twenty to thirty seconds.

Lunge Stretches

For lunges, begin in a standing position and thrust your right leg out in front of you as far as you can manage, with most of your weight resting on your right leg and foot. Your right leg should not be bent beyond a ninety-degree angle. Your left leg should be extended as far as possible directly behind you. In effect, you should now look as though you are preparing to reach out to pick up a baseball grounder or hit a sharply angled tennis ball.

Now, slide your left foot back, inch by inch, until you feel tension through your groin, upper legs, and buttock muscles. You shouldn't feel pain or discomfort, but you should sense that your muscles and tendons are being exposed to a good stretch. Hold this position for twenty to thirty seconds. Then, perform the same movements with your left leg thrust forward and your right leg extended to the rear.

This particular stretch saved one of my middle-aged patients considerable discomfort—if not a bad muscle tear—as the following illustration shows.

The Preventive Power of a Targeted Stretch

At one time in his life, "Peter" played a great deal of squash, which requires movements similar to the lunge stretch as the player runs back and forth on an enclosed court and reaches for fast-moving balls.

But he then quit the sport for about a year and pursued other forms of exercise that didn't require those kinds of movement. Mostly, he engaged in jogging and cycling, with some strength training tossed into the mix every week.

After this one-year hiatus, Peter was invited to play squash again by a friend, and he jumped into the game as though he had competed in the sport just the day before. Unfortunately, his body wasn't up to the task. Before he was finished with the first game, he felt one of his buttock muscles—the gluteus maximus—give way. He didn't suffer a full-fledged muscle tear, but he did have to stop playing, and he had to avoid all forms of exercise for a full ten days before the muscle healed and the pain allowed him to resume his regular aerobic running routine.

This experience impressed Peter with the need to incorporate the lunge stretch into his daily routine, primarily because the movements mimicked quite closely the same squash shot that had immobilized him. After only a couple of weeks, he became so flexible that he was able to do the lunge stretches with the one leg extended so far behind him that he could touch the rear knee on the floor. Also, he purposely put extra pressure on the buttock muscles in an attempt to prepare them for his next squash match.

About nine months later, he was invited to play again, and this time he was physically ready. His targeted stretching routine had conditioned his legs and buttocks so well, both for strength and flexibility, that he made it through five games without a problem.

Peter's experience points to some important principles about

. . . .

exercise in general and stretching in particular. First, the older you get, the more important it is to design your fitness routine wisely, so that your muscles and ligaments will be prepared for any challenge you can imagine. When you're younger, your body is more resilient and preparation for a physical challenge is less necessary. But when you move beyond about age forty, fitness preparation is the name of the game.

Second, stretching must be a part of every complete fitness program. Without flexibility, you won't be able to engage effectively in a wide variety of youthful activities. You'll lack range of motion, and you'll be more vulnerable to injury.

Finally, stretching is essential because it often provides strength training as well as greater flexibility. Note Peter's experience: he not only was able to stretch for the ball, he also had developed the muscle power in his buttocks to move as the game required.

The above stretches are the bare minimum, but they should prepare you for most of the challenges you will encounter to your flexibility. You are certainly free to add others to your program—such as the routines I've described in my previously mentioned books.

Also, there is no commandment that says you must do these the first thing in the morning. You may prefer to do them at the end of your workday, perhaps as part of a warm-up program just before you do a more strenuous aerobic or strength workout.

Doing one or more of these stretches as part of a pick-me-up targeting strategy during the day can be an effective way to overcome feelings of fatigue or achiness. (For an example of how a pick-me-up can work in practice, see Diane's story in Chapter 1.)

THE CROSS-TRAINING CONCEPT

At this point you may be wondering, *How can I possibly design a fitness program that will include every element of this targeting trilogy? I have only twenty-four hours a day, and most of those have to be spent at work or with my family.*

In many ways, cross-training is the answer to your dilemma.

Simply stated, this concept involves the inclusion of several different types of fitness activities in your program each week so that you'll be able to condition many parts of your body, protect yourself against injury, and keep your interest level as high as possible.

One of the biggest problems with most exercise programs is that people get bored. Unless you are by nature a person who loves solitude and repetition, chances are you'll lose interest in a regimen that includes only running or jogging over the same course day in and day out, week after week. The same is true with swimming or other individual endurance sports.

Even if you are an avid tennis or basketball player, with the advantage of being reinforced in your regimen by other players, it's easy to lose interest after months or years of the same activity. That's where cross-training comes in.

Suppose, for instance, that during the course of a given week, you devote a total of three hours of conditioning to several different activities. You might spend an hour playing tennis, a half hour jogging or swimming on your own, a half hour walking with your spouse, and an hour doing strength and flexibility work.

Such a regimen offers several major advantages. First of all, there is enough variety to keep you from getting bored. Second, your motivation is likely to remain high because you're mixing solitary activities (jogging and swimming) with exercise that involves contact with other people (tennis and walking). Third, you're exercising different muscle groups—and thus achieving better whole-body fitness.

In particular, the variety exposes you to the entire trilogy of basic fitness that we've been talking about in this chapter. You achieve bone-building benefits with striking exercises such as tennis and jogging (and perhaps your strength work, if you are concentrating on low-repetition, heavy-resistance weight lifting).

You are strengthening a wide variety of specific muscle groups through the striking exercises, as well as through the swimming and strength work. Also, you're developing endurance through the striking sports, jogging, tennis, and walking. Finally, the flexibility training is helping you retain a youthful range of motion.

Stamina Strategy
Does Training for One Sport Help Condition You for Another?

Specificity in training is essential to excelling at any sport—and that means bringing certain muscle groups and skills to the highest level of performance by doing only exercise that focuses on those specific areas.

But there is evidence that there is a "transfer effect" between activities and sports. Also, for the recreational athlete, cross-training may be the best preparation for overall fitness and for avoiding injury.

A report in the *Journal of Applied Physiology* (Nov. 1988; 65[5]: pp. 2285–90), for instance, showed that heavy-resistance training to increase leg-muscle strength could help highly trained cyclists and runners improve their performance. The researchers from the University of Illinois supervised strength training three days per week for ten weeks, while the cyclists and runners were also pursuing their endurance work.

After ten weeks, the leg strength of all the athletes had increased by an average of 30 percent, and their short-term endurance (for four to eight minutes) increased by 11 to 13 percent. In addition, bicycle riders increased their long-term cycling time from seventy-one to eighty-five minutes after the strength training. The runners, however, didn't experience a similar long-term improvement in their aerobic power.

The researchers concluded that adding heavy-resistance training to an endurance regimen didn't have any negative effects on aerobic performance. They also noted that certain types of endurance performance—especially those requiring the use of "fast-twitch fibers," such as cycling—could be improved with strength work.

Another facet of the benefits of cross-training emerged in a November 1994 report in *Sports Medicine* (Vol. 18, No. 5, pp.

330–9). Researchers from the University of Tennessee at Knoxville found some transfer of aerobic training effects between sports. Specifically, they discovered that there is a noticeable benefit for other endurance sports when running is used as the cross-training mode. The aerobic power developed by swimming, however, displayed only a minimal transfer of training effects.

In any event, the researchers concluded that for the general population, cross-training may be highly beneficial in terms of overall fitness. Also, they said, cross-training may be quite helpful during periods when an athlete is rehabilitating from physical injury or psychological fatigue from his principal sport.

DESIGNING YOUR PERSONAL TARGETING GUIDE

You now have many of the tools required to begin to design your own targeting guide—the specific set of programs that will help you recover and maintain the highest levels of youthful vigor and energy.

First, you understand the importance of the targeting trilogy—or the three key elements of striking, strengthening, and stretching, which must be part of any power of youth program. Unless you prepare your bones, muscles, and endurance systems, you can never approach the high levels of energy and vigor that you enjoyed when you were much younger. On the other hand, if you do incorporate the trilogy into your life, you can begin to regain your lost vigor and other powers.

In addition, you've seen through the examples of Diane in Chapter 1 and Peter in this chapter, as well as a variety of scientific findings, how you can deal with other specific problems, such as getting more energy in the morning or preparing for a sport that you may play only occasionally.

As our discussion unfolds in the following pages, you'll find other specific illustrations of how targeting principles have worked in a wide variety of different situations. But of course, it's impossible for me to lay down a precise blueprint for each individual reader. Designing your particular targeting strategies must ultimately be your responsibility.

But if you begin with the targeting trilogy, make regular use of the Cooper Energy Scale presented in the following chapter, and study the specific examples of targeting in the boxes and other highlighted sections throughout this book, you'll soon discover new sources of vigor, optimism, and energy.

In many respects, this chapter is the fulcrum of the entire book— the basic reference point that supports and balances all the other advice and information. You'll almost certainly find that from time to time, as you continue to fine-tune your personal targeting strategies, you'll need to refer back to the principles and strategies we've discussed here.

But before you can move forward and take meaningful steps to infuse more energy, vigor, and optimism in your life, you have to know where you stand. Just how energetic are you? What are your areas of weakness? Where do you need to focus your targeting strategies to achieve the best effect?

To answer these questions, evaluate your current physical, emotional, and spiritual status according to the Cooper Energy Scale.

3
. . . .

Measuring Your Staying Power on the Cooper Energy Scale

To develop an effective targeting program, you first must measure the current state of your personal energy levels as accurately as possible. In other words, you need a personal energy gauge to check your personal vim and vigor, much as you have a needle on the instrument panel of your car to check your gasoline level. With such a tool, you'll be in a good position to identify major energy weaknesses, specific areas where you lack the strength and stamina to carry on an effective life.

To help you perform this self-assessment, I've devised a ten-point scale, the Cooper Energy Scale, reminiscent of the Borg perceived exertion scale used at the Cooper Clinic and other treadmill testing sites. But there's a major difference between the two approaches. The Borg method focuses on physical fatigue during a specific exercise session, whereas my energy scale is designed to measure a much broader set of factors.

As you'll see in the following section, the Cooper Energy Scale measures your total energy levels on a given day, including your physical, emotional, and even spiritual status. This scale is based on a variety of scientific findings showing strong physiologic, emotional, and spiritual bases for total personal energy—including the resilience that's necessary to support an upbeat, optimistic, youthful attitude toward life.

Now, here is an explanation of the energy scale and some suggestions about how you can use it regularly to the best effect.

THE COOPER ENERGY SCALE: WHAT IT IS AND HOW TO USE IT

As I mentioned earlier, this scale is a prime example of a youth booster—one of those key targeting strategies that will help you regain the power of youth. First, take a quick look at the energy scale. Then we'll discuss how you can make the best use of it.

COOPER ENERGY SCALE

Energy/ Comfort Level	Flexibility	Freedom from Pain	Strength/ Muscle Stamina	Aerobic Endurance	Emotional Status	Spiritual Health
Zero						
Very Low						
Low						
Low Moderate						
Moderate						
High Moderate						
Optimal for Most Tasks						
High						
Very High						
Peak						

Purpose of the Energy Scale

This scale has been designed to provide you with a daily—or even hourly—"snapshot" of your energy levels in several important categories of your life.

The chart requires you to make a subjective evaluation of your sense of well-being in terms of your energy and comfort levels in six specific areas of your life. Some are physical, and others are emotional or spiritual. By doing this self-assessment on a regular basis, you'll be able to pinpoint problem areas—which you'll then be in a position to treat or correct with specific targeting techniques.

Consider buying a spiral notebook or setting up a separate document on your word processor to keep track of your energy levels in different categories. Use the scale printed in this book as a kind of template to guide you as you are making entries.

For example, on today's page you might write, "Flexibility—low moderate," specifying which parts of your body are particularly stiff. Next you might enter, "Emotional Status—optimal," this time noting any areas that could cause problems.

The best approach is to do evaluations at least once a week—and preferably more often—using each of the six categories. Each set of entries should be dated so that after a few months or years, you can look back over your self-assessments and pick up trends or stubborn problems that don't seem to go away.

How to Interpret Specific Categories on the Scale

Energy/Comfort Level. The left-hand column, entitled "Energy/ Comfort Level," contains a ten-point scale, from zero energy or comfort, to peak energy or comfort. The first four levels reflect a subpar sense of well-being or vigor. In other words, if you find you are at any of these levels in flexibility, endurance, emotional power, or spiritual health, you clearly need to find a targeting strategy that will help you raise your energy or comfort level.

If you are in either of the next two levels on the Energy/ Comfort Level column—the moderate or high-moderate range—you probably are functioning adequately, but you could still make good use of a targeting strategy.

The seventh level, "optimal for most tasks," means that you're able to handle most occupational, family, recreational, or other personal challenges that come your way. Targeting techniques may help you raise your energy levels to exceptional heights, but they aren't required for you to lead a full and productive life.

The top three levels usually apply only to those who are:

- exceptionally fit physically, emotionally, and spiritually
- relatively young and healthy
- gifted genetically with unusual amounts of vigor, optimism, strength, or endurance

Flexibility. When you're using the Cooper Energy Scale, you should be systematic in evaluating yourself in each of the six categories, beginning with the first column, labeled "Flexibility."

Here, you should test just how flexible you feel in different parts of your body, beginning at the top and going right to the bottom! In other words, you might first check your shoulders and neck. Ask yourself, "Does my neck feel stiff as I move my head from the right to the left, or forward and backward?"

If you identify a problem, describe it in your spiral notebook or your word processing document. Then continue your checkup, evaluating the rest of your body—such as your trunk (how it feels to bend sideways); your lower back (how it feels to try touching your toes); or your Achilles tendon, lower leg, and ankle.

When you've finished your flexibility assessment, move on to the next column—the degree to which you are in pain.

Freedom from Pain. At first, doing this evaluation according to the "Zero" to "Peak" scale may seem a little confusing. But any difficulties should disappear if you keep in mind that we're talking here about *freedom* from pain, not pain itself.

So if you have frequent but not debilitating lower back pains, or headaches, or some other such discomfort, your freedom from pain will probably be somewhere in the low to low-moderate range. On the other hand, if your pain is debilitating—such as headaches that require you to lie down until they pass—you may be in the zero to very low range. Those who are generally without pain will most likely register their feelings in the high-moderate to optimal range.

As with the flexibility entries, be as specific as you can with your pain evaluations. Details will not only help you keep precise track of your own condition, they will also give you a valuable record to help your physician render a diagnosis and prescribe any necessary treatment.

Strength/Muscle Stamina. Your subjective judgments in this area should focus on such issues as a perceived inability to perform certain strength- or stamina-oriented tasks that you could perform rather easily when you were younger.

Muscle strength refers to the maximum capacity of a muscle to lift a heavy load one time. The stronger you are, the more you can lift in a single effort. For example, suppose you can do a bench press one time with eighty pounds, but you can't do two repetitions. This performance reflects the maximum strength of your muscles that are involved in a bench press—including pectorals (chest muscles) and triceps (muscles on the backs of the arms).

Muscle stamina, also called *muscle endurance*, refers to the ability of a particular set of muscles to perform repetitive or sustained movements with loads that are less than the maximum you can lift. The more times you can lift a submaximal load, the more muscle stamina or endurance you have. Also, the longer you can hold a weight in a certain position, the more muscle stamina you possess. This particular ability to keep a set of muscles contracted for a given period of time is also known as *isometric strength*.

Assume, for instance, that you can raise a set of dumbbells upward in a curling motion from the front of your body up to your chest and back down again twelve times, and a friend can perform the same movements ten times. In this case, you have demonstrated that you have more muscle endurance with that particular weight than she does.

In another variation, imagine that you grasp a horizontal bar and begin to hang suspended from it by your hands, without allowing your feet to touch the ground. The longer you can hang, the more muscle endurance (isometric strength) you have in your hands, arms, and shoulders—at least for performing this particular task.

Other measures of muscle endurance may involve everyday tasks at work, around the house, or in recreational settings. For example, do you find you have trouble carrying a medium-size suitcase from the car rental counter to the airline ticket counter, whereas you could do this rather easily five or ten years ago?

Or do your hands and arms become tired when you type or play the piano for a few minutes now even though you could go for an hour a few years ago?

Or do your calf muscles begin to tighten up and tire after a short period of ballroom dancing or a casual game of volleyball when you wouldn't have given such an activity a second thought when you were younger?

In each of these situations, you are showing how much, or how little, muscle stamina you possess for the particular task in question.

When you make entries on the energy scale about your level of muscle strength or stamina on a given day, you should be specific. In other words, identify the particular muscle or muscle group, and describe as precisely as possible the weakness or inadequacy you are experiencing.

Being quite specific in your recording is especially important with this column because there is usually a great deal you can do through targeting techniques to correct a particular deficiency.

For example, if you have started to travel more and you notice you can't carry a heavy suitcase as far as you once could, the answer may be simply to include extra weight training in your workouts. One possibility would be to do shoulder shrugs with a barbell or dumbbells.

This exercise involves standing up straight and holding the weight with your arms at your sides or in front of the lower part of your body. To do the exercise, you just shrug your shoulders in a rolling motion. One roll constitutes one repetition. Typically, you would use a weight that would allow you to do eight consecutive repetitions. Over the course of a few sessions, you should raise your repetitions to twelve. After you get accustomed to doing twelve repetitions, add a set, another group of eight repetitions. After you can do two or three sets, add extra weights and begin again at one set of eight repetitions.

If you don't have a barbell or dumbbells, you might rely on your creative instincts and devise an even more specific targeting exercise. First, you might get a couple of old suitcases. Then pack enough books in them to simulate a typical heavy suitcase that you have to carry. Finally, walk around the room or your house for a few minutes with one of the suitcases in each hand.

The purpose of having two suitcases instead of one is twofold: first of all, you'll be able to strengthen both sides of your body—and develop the ability to shift a heavy case in the airport from one arm to the other. Second, a basic principle of effective and safe exercise is balance. If you load up one side of your body with heavy weights, the risks increase of hurting your back or pulling a muscle.

Repeat this suitcase exercise two or three times a week for a couple of weeks. Then gradually increase the amount of time you walk by a few minutes. Before long, you'll find that your ability to carry a heavy suitcase over a lengthy period of time will increase significantly. Not only that, the strength and stamina of your "suitcase-carrying" muscles will prepare you to perform other similar tasks, such as carrying heavy groceries or department store bags.

What Influence Do Physical Strength and Stamina Have on Job Fatigue?

The amount of end-of-day fatigue and task strain—physical stress involving specific job assignments—were evaluated in terms of the physical fitness of individual nurses' physical fitness in a 1995 Japanese study.

The study, conducted by the Research Center of Health, Physical Fitness and Sports at Nagoya University, Aichi,

Japan, involved ninety-nine nurses, ages twenty to forty-nine, who were employed at social welfare facilities.

Overall, the researchers found that fatigue complaint rates at the end of a typical workday were about the same for all age-groups, varying from 35 to 38 percent of the participants. Also, four of the twenty-one tasks done by the nurses triggered complaints of strain at rates greater than 50 percent. These high-complaint tasks included nursing seriously ill patients, nursing patients who needed the assistance of medical devices, bathing care, and changing diapers of incontinent patients.

What role did the physical condition of the nurses play in their fatigue and muscle strain?

First of all, those who complained most of fatigue at the end of the day displayed low levels of arm power and cardiovascular endurance, according to the fitness tests they took. Also, complaints about muscle strain were significantly higher in a low-arm-power group that had been doing three particular tasks: nursing seriously ill patients, nursing patients who needed the assistance of devices, and changing diapers.

Finally, complaints about strains suffered after three tasks—nursing patients who needed devices, bathing care, and changing diapers—were significantly higher in a group with low cardiovascular endurance.

The researchers concluded that building arm strength, increasing overall stamina, and alleviating the strains of particular tasks would help reduce excessive fatigue in nurses. (See *Sangyo Eiseigaku Zasshi*, July 1995; 37[4]: pp. 227–33.)

Aerobic Endurance. The best way to measure your precise aerobic power, or cardiovascular endurance, is to take an exercise stress test. This involves having an electrocardiogram taken while you exercise to exhaustion on a treadmill or stationary bicycle. The longer you can exercise under these conditions, the greater your aerobic power. (For a more detailed description of this test, see my book *Can Stress Heal?* [Thomas Nelson Publishers, 1998], p. 219.)

While a well-run stress test can often pick up abnormalities in the heart and should be an integral part of any complete physical exam, the purpose of the energy scale is different. The idea here is to do a series of *subjective* spot checks on your aerobic capacity or endurance at particular times on particular days.

For example, you may have found yourself running out of steam while you were walking in a shopping mall. Or you may have started to huff and puff when you joined a friend for an infrequent game of tennis. Perhaps a hike in the woods with the family on a weekend holiday or a vacation may have tired you out more than it did your companions.

After you have made a number of entries, you should look over your self-evaluations in an effort to determine trends. This survey should help you answer a variety of important questions:

- Is my endurance often lower than that of other people when I go on an outing?
- Do I tend to be about average in terms of my fatigue levels and my ability to "keep up with the crowd" when I'm touring on a holiday?
- Am I usually able to walk faster and farther than my companions, and do I typically end such outings with plenty of energy left over?

Answering such questions will help you evaluate yourself fairly accurately over months or even years in terms of aerobic endurance. Having this broader picture of your capabilities—including any tendency to lose energy or strength in recent years—will enable you to pinpoint areas of weakness that targeting techniques can help you overcome.

For example, one middle-aged woman, "Anne," was referred to our offices because of complaints about fatigue, low energy levels, and bouts with mild depression. Her aerobic capacity was so limited that she was unable to walk around a normal city block without stopping to rest.

Anne's friends, who liked to chat while strolling outdoors, were willing to accept her lack of endurance up to a point. But when they became deeply involved in some conversations and wanted to keep walking and talking for a longer distance than normal, they sometimes lost patience with her.

Fortunately, Anne's problems were easily remedied. We put her on a moderate walking regimen, which required her to walk at a reasonably brisk pace a half hour a day, five days a week. Before one month had passed, Anne had increased her endurance to the point that she felt she was being held back by the slow pace of her friends!

Furthermore, her periods of depression disappeared altogether, apparently as a result of the release of endorphins during her exercise.

Though she was not using my energy scale, Anne had done the next-best thing: she had identified her problem quite accurately—and had accepted a highly effective targeting solution.

Emotional Status. In this column, you should evaluate both your personal emotional status and the state of your relationships. Relationships might include several categories, such as family members, friends, or colleagues and supervisors at work. Because of the multiple nature of entries you might make in this column, you will often find yourself making notations in several boxes.

In other words, if you personally are feeling quite anxious because of some problem at work, you might rank yourself low in the Emotional Status category to indicate the state of your personal emotions. On the other hand, if you are feeling a significant surge of well-being in your marriage or family relationships, you might record this fact with a check in the "optimal" space. Finally, if some of your friendships are going through some slightly rocky moments, you might indicate that in the "low moderate" area.

Often, however, you'll probably find that the quality of your emotions is similar right across the board—for your emotional life and your relationships. So if you personally are feeling depressed, the chances are your interactions with your family and friends won't be going too well either. And if you are feeling cheerful and optimistic, your attitude is likely to be reflected in positive relationships with others.

Spiritual Health. In some ways, this column is the most difficult to define or grasp because of the difficulty of giving a general definition of the word *spiritual.* In general, what I am referring to here is the state of the inner being, often referred to in religious terms as the *spirit* or the *soul.* Obviously, religious and philosophical factors, including one's view of God and the nature of the human relationship to Him, are essential to this definition.

The inner spiritual life is generally understood to be related to, but still distinct from, the emotional life. In other words, it's possible to experience joy on an emotional plane when a child achieves a significant goal at school. At the same time, there may be a different sense of joy—one that can only be described as "spiritual"—when the child experiences a significant breakthrough in establishing a deeper relationship with God, such as through a personal renewal or a conversion experience.

Those who affirm an established religious tradition will most likely understand exactly what I mean. For example, as a Christian, I know that my spiritual health is directly dependent upon how well I am nurturing my relationship with God. I might ask myself such questions as these:

- How regularly am I praying?
- How often do I study my Bible?
- Am I experiencing inner peace—or the "peace that passes understanding," a deep tranquillity of soul that transcends mere emotional definitions?
- Am I developing strong relationships with others who profess spiritual beliefs similar to or compatible with mine?
- Is my spiritual life having a beneficial impact on the world

around me—including my work environment and my various friends and acquaintances?

These are just a few of the issues that you might consider as you evaluate your spiritual health on the energy scale. And remember, scientific research is increasingly demonstrating a strong link between emotional and physical health on the one hand and spiritual disciplines, such as prayer, on the other. (For more on this connection, see the "Spiritual Monitor" discussion in Chapter 5. Also, there is a variety of references linking prayer and healing under the index entry *prayer* in *Can Stress Heal?*)

In the same vein, a connection is being recognized increasingly in medical circles between such spiritual disciplines and your personal health and energy levels. (The accompanying box provides a preliminary illustration.)

How Doctors Can Develop the Stamina to Handle Difficult Health Care Challenges

A comprehensive 1994 review article, produced at the hospice at the Texas Medical Center in Houston, described the personal resources a physician needs to manage the symptoms of patients with advanced cancer.

According to the weight of scientific literature, to do an effective job of helping patients with advanced cancer through the final difficulties of life, the physician must attend to his own spiritual, psychosocial, and physical needs. When the physician is prepared both inwardly and outwardly, the author of this study says, the patients will be in a much stronger position to complete their lives in the place of their choosing, with the comfort and support needed to finish business, deal with strained relationships, and confront the mysteries of life and death. (See *Seminal Oncology*, Dec. 1994; 21[6]: pp. 748–53.)

FINE-TUNING YOUR EVALUATION ON THE ENERGY SCALE

Now that you have a general sense of what the Cooper Energy Scale is and how it works, let's turn to some specific "energy sappers" that can cause you to turn in a low score on the scale. They include:

- general bad stress
- depression
- inadequate sleep
- a pessimistic attitude
- dehydration

These factors, along with the nine causes of youth drain described in Chapter 4, comprise the most important indicators of what may be causing you to feel fatigued, depressed, or otherwise emotionally, physically, or spiritually out of sorts.

If you score below the moderate range in any of the columns on the scale, you should immediately check to see if one of the following energy-sapping factors is present in your life. The chances are, you'll immediately be able to identify the cause of your problem. Then you'll be in a position to devise an effective targeting strategy to eliminate your low-voltage energy condition.

BAD STRESS: THE MAJOR REASON FOR LOW-VOLTAGE ENERGY

When I score below the moderate level on any of the six columns on the energy scale, I immediately go through a mental checklist of areas in my life that may be producing bad stress. There is such a thing as good stress. Good stress involves a healthy internal response to the pressures and tensions in life, which can cause us to perform better and reach levels of achievement that we never dreamed possible. In effect, good stress enhances personal energy levels and enables us to keep going beyond our usual limits of stamina and strength.

Bad stress, in contrast, refers to a negative response to outer or inner pressures, which leads to a depletion of personal stores of energy. I often tell my patients, "You usually experience bad stress for one of two possible reasons: either you're in a situation that you shouldn't be in, or you're in a situation that you can't get out of. The best response to the first situation is to avoid it. The best response to the second is to determine immediately how to take control."

Here are some of the most recent findings about how uncontrolled bad stress can sap your power of youth and your good health—and some suggestions for learning how to exert control over various problems that produce this negative stress:

The Broad Impact of Chronic Stress

A 1998 study confirmed that chronic stress can trigger harmful physical responses and interact with destructive lifestyle habits. This dynamic typically promotes such damaging physiological changes as insulin resistance, heart disease, memory loss, immune system dysfunction, and decreased bone mineral density.

The report, published in the *New England Journal of Medicine* and summarized in a January 25, 1998, article in *The Washington Post*, noted that there are eight major "markers"—or risk factors—for stress-related damage. These include high blood pressure, high blood sugar, high cholesterol, high levels of the adrenal hormone cortisol, and excess abdominal fat.

The author of the report, a researcher from Rockefeller University in New York City, affirmed the well-known fact that the body responds to stressful situations by producing extra amounts of the adrenal hormones. When the threat recedes, the hormone production is supposed to be inactivated—but this doesn't always happen.

Those who continue to produce excess adrenal hormones after a threat or stressful situation has disappeared may experience the various physical problems and diseases mentioned above.

What is the targeting solution to this problem?

The report suggests that those who don't handle stress well—and who experience increased blood pressure, anxiety, and other signs of bad stress—should focus on learning coping skills, such as how to relax. Also, because there is a negative interaction between bad stress and bad health habits, they should choose a low-fat diet, quit smoking, and embark on a regular exercise program.

In addition, the report says, those who aren't handling stress well should work at improving their social relationships and avoid isolation. Another important area to evaluate is the work environment: those who lack adequate control over their job assignments are much more vulnerable to developing the symptoms of bad stress.

The Latest on How Bad Stress Can Hurt Your Heart

According to a report in the December 2, 1997, issue of *Circulation*, a failure to handle stress well may be a factor in damaging vessels and developing blocked arteries.

Researchers from the University of Pittsburgh evaluated how the blood pressures of more than twenty-six hundred Finnish men, ages forty-two to sixty, responded to mental and motor-skills tests when the men were under stress. The tests required that the subjects perform at levels of difficulty that limited them to an accuracy rate of 60 percent.

Follow-up studies done over an eight- to ten-year period showed that the 20 percent who reacted most negatively to the mental stress tests (with higher spikes in blood pressure) had thicker carotid arteries than the 20 percent who had the least negative reaction.

The carotid arteries are the two main arteries in the neck that channel blood to the brain. Generally speaking, a tendency to develop blockages in the carotid arteries indicates a tendency to develop atherosclerosis, the buildup of plaque in the arteries, which can lead to a stroke.

The researchers speculated that frequent and prolonged periods of elevated blood pressure during stressful situations may damage the artery linings or cause release of adrenal hormones that can lead to the depositing of plaque in the vessel walls.

Another interesting finding of the study was that the blood pressure readings of men under age fifty-five were most likely to surge with stress, and these men were most likely to develop thicker artery walls.

The Power of Stress-Reduction Techniques

At an October 1997 conference sponsored by the American Medical Association, researchers from Duke University Medical Center reported that stress-reduction techniques could lower the risk of heart attacks by 74 percent.

Their study, which was scheduled for publication in the *Archives of Internal Medicine*, involved 107 patients who experienced impaired blood flow to the heart during mental stress tests or as they wore heart monitors during daily activities.

To check the benefits of stress-reduction techniques, the patients were divided into three groups. One group took a four-month stress management program. They first learned how to recognize their own responses to stressful situations. Then they practiced relaxation techniques such as meditative strategies to calm the mind, biofeedback conditioning, and strategies to change the way they viewed stressful situations.

For example, instead of saying to themselves, "This person is really irritating me," they might work to express that reaction in more positive, constructive terms, such as, "I wonder why this person is so unhappy? Is there anything I can do to help?"

A second group in the study engaged in a four-month exercise program, and the third group just received normal care from their physicians.

The results: of the total number of patients in the study, twenty-two suffered at least one cardiac event within five years of undergoing their treatment programs. But the cardiac problems plagued only three in the stress management group, whereas seven in the exercise group and twelve in the routine medical care group had heart trouble.

Experts commenting on the report noted that among the eleven million Americans with heart disease, an estimated 50 to 60 percent develop ischemia (reduced blood and oxygen flow to tissues such as the heart) when under emotional stress, and 40 to 50 percent suffer from ischemia during their normal daily activities. (See also the Associated Press report, Oct. 26, 1997, and the Scripps Howard News Service report, Oct. 20, 1997.)

The Crisis of Job Control

Increasingly, a lack of control on the job is emerging as a primary source of debilitating stress—and a major threat to youthful vigor.

A study published in July 1997 in the British medical journal *Lancet* followed almost seventy-four hundred women and men in London government jobs for an average of more than five years, between 1985 and 1993.

The researchers found that those who had minimal control over their work responsibilities faced a 50 percent higher risk of suffering from heart disease symptoms than did those in higher positions.

Experts who speculated on the reason for these findings suggested that a lack of control might trigger higher levels of stress hormones, which can elevate the blood levels of fibrinogen, a protein that promotes clotting. In support of this interpretation, the study found that higher blood levels of fibrinogen were associated with low job control.

This chemical action, along with other hormonal and immune system changes, may damage the coronary arteries that channel blood to the heart. (See also *The Wall Street Journal*, July 25, 1997, and the related Associated Press report published on the same date.)

Does the boss, who typically has more control over his responsibilities, ever confront control-related stress?

In an ironic twist, the Onset Study released on March 19, 1998, at a conference in Santa Fe, New Mexico, reported on work-stress research conducted at forty-five hospitals across the United States. According to researchers from Beth Israel Deaconess Medical Center in Boston, the study provides strong evidence that managers who fire someone run double the usual risk of a heart attack during the week following the dismissal.

The greatest danger to the heart occurred for those who had to do the firing while working under a high-pressure deadline, according to a Beth Israel Deaconess researcher. (See also the Associated Press report, published March 20, 1998.)

A Link Between Stress and Breast Cancer?

Clearly, cancer is one of the most devastating energy sappers confronting us today. Sometimes, there may be little we can do to avoid this disease, but it is possible to reduce the statistical risk by reducing stress.

Breast cancer is a case in point. In a study published on January 7, 1998, in the *Journal of the National Cancer Institute*, researchers from Ohio State University reported that breast cancer patients with the most anxiety had the lowest levels of "natural killer" (NK) cells—part of the immune defenses that control cancer cells and fight infection. Specifically, women with high levels of stress had 20 to 30 percent fewer natural killer cells, which have the power to kill cancer cells.

Researchers noted that the study, which involved 116 women who had undergone surgery for breast cancer, was only the first step in exploring the link between stress and breast cancer. The next step is to do further investigation to see if stress-reduction strategies can help more of the cancer patients recover successfully. (See also the Associated Press report, published Jan. 7, 1998.)

Eye-Opener
Should You Blame Blue Monday?

Research by Dr. James Muller, chief of cardiology at the University of Kentucky, Lexington, determined years ago that heart attacks tend to strike on Monday mornings. Furthermore, the Framingham Heart Study determined in research released in 1995 that strokes also peak on Monday mornings. Recent research at the Baltimore Veterans Administration

Medical Center has shown that 21 percent of heart-rhythm disturbances strike on Monday mornings—a figure that is twice the weekend rate.

So to reduce your risk of these cardiovascular events, should you call in sick on Mondays?

Actually, according to researchers in this area, a more productive approach involves a two-step strategy.

First, take steps to lower your overall risk of heart attacks and strokes, such as exercising regularly, quitting smoking, eating a heart-healthy low-fat diet, controlling your blood pressure, and lowering your cholesterol.

Then, if you can ease into your Mondays in a less stressful way, by all means do so. For example, to get your blood flowing on this first day of the workweek, you might try some of the eye-opener exercises and stretching routines described in Chapters 1 and 2. Also, if possible, consider scheduling light, undemanding work and meetings for Mondays. The tough, potentially confrontational or highly stressful assignments should be placed in the middle part of the week.

For those who are cardiac patients, some medical intervention may be required to reduce the Monday threat, such as:

- taking beta-blocker drugs to control heartbeat irregularities and lower the chances of another heart attack
- taking an aspirin a day, under a physician's supervision

Fortunately, however, for those with no history of heart problems, the risk of Monday health problems is minimal. In fact, some experts have estimated that the average person's risk of a cardiovascular problem on Mondays versus other days may go up from about one in a million to two in a million! (See *The Wall Street Journal*, Sept. 30, 1996, p. B1.)

Four More Energy Sappers

As you are trying to evaluate yourself as precisely as possible on the energy scale, you shouldn't stop your self-assessment after you've identified the major stresses in your life. As I mentioned earlier, there are four other important factors that can sap the energy of youth: depression, inadequate sleep, pessimism, and dehydration.

Here is some of the latest evidence on these factors—and some suggestions about how you can manage them.

Depression

If you are feeling depressed, the chances are you will score below moderate on several columns of the Energy Scale, including emotional status, spiritual health, and probably some of the physical tests, such as aerobic endurance.

Clinical depression plagues about one-fifth of Americans, according to a January 1997 report from the American Medical Association. Peter Harnisch, a pitcher for the New York Mets, revealed that he had been placed on the disabled list because of this problem. His symptoms included interrupted sleep, poor appetite, and physical exhaustion. (See *The New York Times*, May 1, 1997, p. A21.)

High levels of despair or hopelessness have also been linked to atherosclerosis. According to a report published in the August 1997 issue of *Arteriosclerosis, Thrombosis and Vascular Biology*, researchers determined that those who expressed a high amount of despair had a 20 percent greater chance of developing atherosclerosis over a four-year period. The investigators noted that this was the same magnitude of increased risk that is seen when comparing a pack-a-day smoker with a nonsmoker.

The important thing about this study was that it showed that a sense of hopelessness can affect the arteries early in the process of plaque buildup.

The lesson we should derive from this report seems clear. Anyone, of any age, who records a high sense of depression, hopelessness, or despair on the Energy Scale (at or below the low level) should take immediate steps to overcome those feelings or symptoms.

How do you go about this? Sometimes, antidepressant drugs are necessary—and certainly, if a sense of depression continues for more than two straight weeks, you should consult your physician. (For some of the latest information on the issue of medication for depression, see the accompanying box.)

Rx Response
Treating Depression Without Endangering the Heart

In the past, it was considered dangerous for heart patients to be treated for depression because certain antidepressants, including a class known as *tricyclics*, might make heart problems worse. All that has apparently changed now with the advent of the new antidepressants known as "selective serotonin reuptake inhibitors." The best known of this new group is the drug Prozac (known generically as *fluoxetine*).

A study published in May 1998 in the *American Journal of Psychiatry* evaluated eighty-seven men and women with an average age of seventy-three who suffered from both severe heart disease and depression. Prozac was given to twenty-seven of the patients, while sixty others received one of the tricyclics, nortriptyline.

During the seven weeks of the evaluation, twelve of the sixty patients on the tricyclics suffered from deteriorating heart conditions. But only one of the Prozac patients had worsening heart problems—and the heart function of several of the Prozac patients actually improved. The researchers cautioned that the study was small and limited, but they did regard the findings as "encouraging." (See "Health Watch," *The New York Times*, June 16, 1998, p. B10.)

On the other hand, if you are plagued mainly by periodic bouts of mild depression, you will probably be able to deal with the problem yourself. Among the most effective ways to overcome the problem: you should consider developing a more optimistic, upbeat attitude, nurturing your spiritual life, and stimulating your creative side. We'll explore these and other responses to hopelessness in Chapter 5.

Inadequate Sleep

Whenever I become tired, the very first factor I evaluate is my "sleep deficit."

Over the years, I've felt that I needed less sleep than most other people. Getting five or six hours a night over a period of months was a typical practice for me, especially when I was younger. Yet I know now, after taking a closer look at both my real needs and the scientific literature, that to function reasonably well, I really need closer to seven hours a night. Furthermore, to be fully rested and at maximum energy levels, it's best if I get a little more or fit a short nap into my day.

So when I'm feeling tired and I glance at that energy scale, the first question that usually comes to mind is this: *Did I get enough shut-eye last night?*

According to a Gallup poll published in June 1997, about one-third of adult Americans feel sleepy during the day. The poll, sponsored by the National Sleep Foundation, found that 6 percent of those surveyed were classified as having severe daytime sleepiness—a condition that could impair their capacity to function safely. Of those who reported they often experience daytime sleepiness, about 40 percent said it interfered with their daily activities. According to the SleepWake Disorders Center at Montefiore Medical Center in New York, falling asleep at the wheel of vehicles causes at least a hundred thousand traffic accidents and fifteen hundred traffic deaths annually.

Symptoms of sleep deprivation include the following, often in this order of occurrence:

- irritability
- excessive fatigue or exhaustion after tasks that would ordinarily present no problem

- headaches
- difficulty dealing with new concepts or creative challenges
- inability to concentrate
- short-term memory loss
- depression and anxiety
- blurred vision
- hallucinations

How can you protect yourself against sleep deprivation and ensure this energy sapper won't rob you of the power of youth? Here are some practical suggestions—classic youth boosters and pick-me-ups—that will help you target and defeat this problem:

Avoid alcohol, caffeine, and smoking. These three substances work against relaxed, sound sleep and prove to be the main obstacles that many people face to a good night's rest. Avoid them, especially just before bedtime.

Establish a firm hour for bedtime. Choose a specific time and discipline yourself to go to bed then, regardless of whether there is a "great TV show" or some other event that is tempting you to stay up.

Break your "worry loops." If you are worried about something at bedtime, you're likely to keep thinking about it when you retire—and it may be an hour or more before you fall asleep. To counter this tendency, here's an effective strategy, which has been suggested by a variety of sleep experts:

Pick a line of a poem, a Bible verse, or some soothing saying and begin to repeat it silently after you turn out the light. If you find your mind wandering, don't fight your lack of concentration. Just turn back easily to the words you've chosen.

This approach, which is in effect a content-oriented form of counting sheep, works consistently for most people. Most likely, you'll never make it past twenty or thirty repetitions before you're sound asleep.

Find time for naps. If you're feeling tired in the middle of the day, there's nothing wrong with closing the door to your office and taking a snooze. But try to limit your nap time to about twenty minutes.

Sleeping much longer in the middle of the day can make you groggy, but limiting yourself to fifteen to twenty minutes can provide a pick-me-up.

Evaluate your sleep environment. If your room is too warm or cold, your bed is too lumpy, or there's too much noise outside the door, you may find yourself fighting a losing battle trying to get to sleep. Targeting responses for these simple but potentially devastating enemies of good sleep include adjusting the room temperature (colder is usually better, so long as you have enough blankets); getting a better mattress; and using earplugs to shut out the noise.

Avoid vigorous exercise within about three hours of bedtime. As important as regular exercise is for your health, a hard, exhausting workout just before bedtime will usually cause you to remain wide-awake well after you turn the lights out. Remember, high-intensity exercise can be a powerful relaxant and energizer when you need a natural tranquilizer or a pick-me-up at the end of the day. But it's not an effective sleep potion. One the other had, a relaxing walk before bedtime may be just as effective as a sleeping pill.

Avoid excessive intake of any beverage just before bedtime. Many people find that as they grow older, they have to get up more often during the night to urinate. For men, the problem may be prostate enlargement; for women, aging itself may reduce bladder control.

To cut down on the number of trips to the bathroom during the night, it's often helpful to avoid that last glass of water, juice, or milk just before bedtime. Also, I recommend that my patients with sleep interruption problems urinate just before they go to bed. This way, their bladders will be as empty as possible before they fall asleep.

A Pessimistic Attitude

If you believe that you will be energetic and youthful on a given day, the chances are that you will indeed possess more vigor. On the other hand, if you begin the day thinking about your aches and pains and fatigue—or anticipating such feelings—your outlook will be precisely the opposite. The odds are excellent that you'll have a below-par day and be forced to make many *low moderate* or lower entries on your energy scale.

What's happening here is sometimes referred to as the "nocebo effect"—or the tendency of a negative belief or attitude to produce a negative health result. This is the other side of the coin of the placebo effect, the positive health benefits that may result from our beliefs.

Dr. Herbert Benson of the Harvard Medical School, who has done considerable research into mind-body interactions, has suggested that our negative attitudes, such as fear, may trigger action in the insular cortex of the brain and lead to ventricular fibrillation (excessively rapid beating of the heart).

Other studies have shown that pessimistic patients may experience reduced blood flow to the heart and greater risk of death than those who are not caught up in negative thinking. Also, negative beliefs have been shown to trigger asthmatic attacks. (From remarks at a November 28, 1995, American Health Foundation conference in New York City.)

In my own practice, I've noticed that those patients who tend to have a pessimistic outlook on life are the most likely to come down with serious health problems, and are also the slowest to recover from an illness.

"Joan," an otherwise healthy forty-five-year-old single professional woman, was constantly complaining about imagined aches and pains. In many ways, she was a classic hypochondriac—so worried about her health that she seemed to have little time to think about anything else.

On a typical morning, she would arise with a slightly stiff back and stiff Achilles tendons. Although this sort of stiffness is common as we age and can usually be alleviated by simple stretching exercises the first thing in the morning, Joan preferred to worry rather than take targeting steps to remedy her situation. Furthermore, as the day wore on, she complained that she increasingly felt physically fatigued and mentally dull.

As it happened, her problems weren't entirely in her mind: she was beginning to get feedback from her senior colleagues that some of her work was unacceptable. Also, she had noticed that she seemed to be getting colds and the flu much more often than when she was younger.

Joan knew she needed medical help to solve this mystery. Among other things, she was afraid that her problem might involve hormonal problems or some chemical imbalance. Home medical guides she was reading suggested that her symptoms might involve a problem with the thyroid gland, a pituitary tumor, or perhaps even a growing brain tumor. Naturally, those prospects frightened her.

After Joan had undergone a thorough checkup, including a wide variety of tests by an endocrinologist, her physician pronounced her basically healthy. But the physician was also wise enough to perceive that most of Joan's difficulties lay in her negative, pessimistic attitudes and expectations.

"You're literally talking and thinking yourself into illness," the doctor said. "What you have to do is to begin to focus on the positive rather than the negative. If you do, I predict that before you know it, you'll start feeling better."

It sounded much too simple to Joan. But she decided to try this approach before she switched doctors. So with the help of the physician and her pastor, she devised what amounted to a short but potent spiritual targeting routine.

The first thing every morning, she would read a short passage from a daily devotional guide or from her Bible. Then she would spend a couple of minutes sitting quietly with her eyes closed and focus on the most uplifting thing she had gleaned from her reading. If negative thoughts—including worries about her health—intruded, she would push them aside and return to her meditation.

After about five minutes of this positive-thinking time, she turned to a specially designed eye-opener routine, a light exercise program that focused mainly on slow stretches for her lower back, hamstring muscles, Achilles tendons, and upper back and arms. She also did a brief set of abdominal crunches (half sit-ups, with knees bent and arms folded in an X across the chest).

As Joan did these exercises, she continued to focus on the positive thoughts that she had used to start her day. In other words, the meditations continued even after the physical activity had begun.

During the day, she occasionally mulled over that first positive thought she had experienced earlier in the morning. The idea here was not to become obsessive or to feel guilty if she forgot to pursue this positive-thinking exercise in every waking moment. Rather, she was attempting to establish a positive mooring for her life—an upbeat, constructive spiritual/psychological pick-me-up to hold on to as the day progressed and the challenges to her good attitude intensified.

Finally, at the end of the day, Joan returned once again to the devotional thoughts that had been her focus when she woke up. She read the same passages and meditated briefly on the Bible verse or other thought that had helped her get started many hours earlier. As she liked to put it, "The circle must be completed."

After a few weeks of this practice, she even began to keep a journal on her growing, positively oriented inner life. If a particular thought had taken on a helpful, practical meaning during the day, she recorded her insight.

For example, one day her special thought was, "Don't let the sun go down on your anger." Coincidentally, she had become very angry with one of her colleagues that day, and they had exchanged some harsh words. Before she had started her "anti-pessimism" program, she would have stewed about the encounter throughout the day and gone home without seeking a resolution. But this time, she made a special point of seeking out her antagonist and taking steps to effect reconciliation.

Sometimes, such an attempt will fail. But more often, making an overture toward peace will help the situation to some extent—and that's what happened in Joan's case.

As you can see, Joan's problem—and the targeting solution she used—went to a deeper cause, far beyond her initial physical and emotional symptoms. Her fundamental problem was a pessimistic spirit that impinged on the health of her emotions and her spiritual life. But by making a more upbeat, positive attitude the centerpiece of her life—and by reinforcing that new attitude with early-morning exercises—she was able to eliminate her physical aches and her flagging energy levels in a matter of a couple of weeks. Also, her efficiency at work returned to the youthful levels that had characterized her performance when she was fifteen years younger.

As simplistic as it may sound to some, the development of an upbeat attitude toward life and of a positive belief system is the cornerstone of good health. Optimism is one of the most powerful antidotes to depression, anxiety, and a host of other emotional ills—not to mention the mental trigger that can lead to relief or cure of many physical maladies. As positive expectations increase, bad stress decreases, the immune system becomes stronger, and overall health tends to improve.

Dehydration

The last big energy sapper that I want to highlight at this point is the failure of most people to drink enough fluids—a problem that will almost always reduce personal drive and vigor and may result in a serious risk to health.

The most dramatic examples of this problem involve health crises faced by older people in Texas and elsewhere during severe heat waves. There's also danger for relatively young and healthy individuals who stay outdoors and perspire copiously while neglecting to replenish their body's fluid supply by drinking enough water or other nonalcoholic, noncaffeinated drinks. The result is often an increased incidence of heat exhaustion (symptoms: profuse sweating, dizziness, clammy skin) or heat stroke (symptoms: hot, dry skin and fever). Heat stroke can cause brain damage or death.

The targeting responses to these problems involve well-known principles of first aid. For heat exhaustion, you should immediately seek a shady or air-conditioned location, sit or lie down, and drink as much water or diluted sports drink as you can handle. Avoid physical activity for the rest of the day, and if symptoms such as dizziness persist, see a physician.

For heat stroke, which is the more dangerous of the two conditions, you should be placed in a shady or air-conditioned location and have cold water or ice applied to your skin to reduce your body temperature. If possible, immerse your body in a cold tub of water; add ice to the water if it's available.

But as I said, these are the most dramatic examples. Subtler—and far more common—problems with dehydration occur every day in most homes and offices throughout the country, as people drink enough to avoid a health crisis but not enough to avoid energy depletion, emotional irritability, constipation, and possibly kidney stones, as the following box explains.

Rx Response
What Is the Link Between Beverages
and Kidney Stones?

Physicians routinely advise their patients with kidney stones to increase their fluid intake as a preventive measure to decrease the risk of the stones recurring in the future. But this advice can become complicated when you begin to distinguish among different types of drinks.

In a 1996 study published in the *American Journal of Epidemiology*, researchers from the Harvard School of Public Health evaluated how twenty-one different beverages impacted the risk of developing kidney stones in a population of more than forty-five thousand men ages forty to seventy-five. Here are some of the rather surprising findings that emerged during six years of follow-up:

The risk of stone formation decreased by the following percentages for each eight-ounce serving of the indicated beverages:

- caffeinated coffee—a 10 percent decrease
- decaffeinated coffee—a 10 percent decrease

- tea—a 14 percent decrease
- beer—a 21 percent decrease
- wine—a 39 percent decrease

The eight-ounce servings of beverages that increased the risk of kidney stones included:

- apple juice—a 35 percent increase
- grapefruit juice—a 37 percent increase

(See *American Journal of Epidemiology*, Feb. 1, 1996; 143[3]: pp. 240–7.)

The results of this study, in which my good friend Dr. Walter Willett participated, were somewhat unexpected because the drinks that we usually think of as presenting health problems, such as those containing caffeine and alcohol, were the "good" drinks. In contrast, the otherwise healthy drinks, apple juice and grapefruit juice, ended up in the "bad" category.

It seems to me that one lesson we can take away from this is that for those with kidney problems, or a family history of stones, apple juice and grapefruit juice should be avoided.

On the other hand, that doesn't mean that it's necessarily a great idea to begin to drink large quantities of caffeine or alcohol. Instead, it seems best to design a balanced nutrition program in consultation with your physician and a qualified dietitian. Such a program should be integrated into all your health needs, as well as your medication regimen.

Most medical experts recommend that you drink at least eight 8-ounce glasses of water or water-equivalent beverages per day (thirteen 8-ounce glasses of water if you engage in sports or other activities that cause you to perspire freely). Examples of hydrating drinks that are about the same as water include fruit juices, sports drinks containing electrolytes and other salts needed by the body, and nonalcoholic and noncaffeinated sodas. Avoid drinks that are carbonated, extremely salty, or very sweet. You want fluids that are as pure as possible. Sometimes, however, a "bad" drink can be disguised as a seemingly helpful drink.

For example, a recent survey sponsored by the International Bottled Water Association and Nutrition Information Center at the New York Hospital-Cornell Medical Center, New York City, revealed that on average, Americans consume 8.5 cups of hydrating beverages per day. By their definition, they included milk as well as water, juices, and caffeine-free drinks. (I omit milk from my list because it requires more digestive activity than the other drinks, so in my view milk and other dairy-related drinks are best classified as foods rather than fluids.)

These findings would have been encouraging except for one big problem: the average person also drank 4.5 cups of caffeinated beverages (such as coffee, tea, and sodas) or alcoholic beverages each day. These fall into the category of dehydrating drinks; they are diuretics, which cause the drinker to urinate more frequently. The end result is a net loss of fluids from the body.

The typical consequences of not drinking enough water—or drinking enough but subtracting from its impact by drinking a dehydrating beverage—include symptoms of mild dehydration. Those with this problem may suffer from grogginess in the morning, dry skin, and generalized fatigue.

According to the researchers at the Nutrition Information Center, a good rule of thumb is to assume that for every cup of coffee or other dehydrating beverage you drink, you should add an extra cup of water. Also, it's important not to wait until you feel thirsty to take a drink. By the time your throat is dry, you'll probably already be a couple of cups behind in your fluid intake. (See *The New York Times*, June 16, 1998, p. B10.)

On the positive side, an increase in your fluid intake can translate into greater physical endurance. One study, published in the *European Journal of Applied Psychology* in 1989 (Vol. 58, No. 5, pp. 481–6), showed how this can work with prolonged cycle exercise.

Researchers from the University Medical School, Aberdeen, Scotland, examined the effects of fluid ingestion on exercise performance. Six male volunteers exercised to exhaustion in a series of tests, at a workload requiring about 70 percent of their physical output. On one of the tests they started off with nothing to drink; on the other tests, they drank a hydrating beverage.

The investigators found that when the six participants exercised without fluids, they lasted for a mean time of 70.2 minutes. In contrast, when they drank a glucose-electrolyte solution, they had more staying power, making it to 90.8 minutes.

But what fluids are best for you? For the best overall health, I stand behind citrus juices, as the next box will explain.

Rx Response
The Curious Case of Citrus

One of the best categories of drinks for getting fluids into your body, along with other important nutrients, is citrus juice. The citrus family includes the orange, grapefruit, lemon, lime, and tangerine.

The health benefits of citrus have been highly touted. They give us anticancer, heart-healthy nutrients, such as vitamin C, bioflavonoids, and folic acid.

The virtues of orange juice, for instance, were highlighted in a 1996 animal study published in *Nutrition and Cancer* (Vol. 26, No. 2, pp. 167–81). Researchers from the University of Western Ontario found that the animals that were given orange juice had a lower number of tumors than a control group, which received no citrus. The investigators concluded that these experiments provide evidence of the anticancer properties of orange juice and indicated that the citrus flavonoids can inhibit the proliferation of human breast cancer cells in a laboratory setting.

But as we saw in the previous box on kidney stones, when you move beyond water, each drink must be evaluated from a medical viewpoint—especially as to how it may interact with your specific health problems and medications.

Grapefruit juice is a case in point. Not only has it been associated with an increase in the incidence of kidney stones, but it's also been linked to some interesting drug interactions. Specifically, a number of studies have shown that drinking grapefruit juice can increase the absorption and concentration—or *bioavailability*—of many drugs in the human body.

According to a review article in the April 1998 issue of *Drug Safety* (Vol. 18, No. 4, pp. 251–72), grapefruit juice can increase blood levels of many drugs by suppressing a key enzyme in the wall of the small intestine. The drugs that are most likely to be taken into the body quickly with grapefruit juice include felodipine (brand name Plendil), nitrendipine, nisoldipine, and saquinavir. Those that are also affected, though less powerfully, include nifedipine (Procardia), nimokipine, verapamil (Calan), cyclosporine (Neoral), midazolam, triazolam (Halcion), and terfenadine (Seldane).

The author of the article cautioned that this list of drugs is incomplete because of a lack of studies on other medications. But he did recommend that patients refrain from drinking grapefruit juice when they are taking one of the drugs that enter the system easily when combined with the citrus drink.

Because so little is known about the impact of grapefruit juice on medications, it's best for anyone on any type of medication to stay away from the drink—unless a study has clearly shown that combining the drug and grapefruit juice is a safe practice.

Now, let's turn to a series of threats in our culture that can undercut the power of youth in anyone, regardless of age. Defeating these dangers—which cause the debilitating, energy-destroying condition that I call *youth drain*—should be a first line of defense for both young and old.

4
·············

Defeating the Threat of Youth Drain

A thirty year old can feel old, just as a seventy year old can feel young. Why is this?

A major reason is that one or more of a series of common negative forces or factors—which comprise what I call youth drain—can rob anyone, of any age, of the vigor, resilience, stamina, and energy of youth. These main causes of youth drain include:

- nagging, recurrent health complaints
- feelings that you are no longer competing at your peak
- tensions caused by time pressures
- the punishing emotional and physical effects of excessive travel, including business travel
- financial worries
- unexpected effects of menopause—both male and female
- frustrations with child rearing
- exhaustion from technology and information overload
- wrong expectations about your health and the aging process

Now, here is a more detailed look at each of these factors—and also some suggestions about how a targeting strategy can become the key to solving the youth drain challenge.

CAUSE 1: NAGGING, RECURRENT HEALTH COMPLAINTS

"Keith," a muscular, athletic real estate agent in his late thirties, had been in the habit since he left college of engaging in demanding cross-training workouts. His regimen featured several exercises that conditioned a wide variety of muscle groups.

Typically, he would bicycle twice a week for an average of twenty miles per outing. Also, he would jog three to four miles at least once a week. On his "off" days, which usually occurred twice a week, he concentrated on doing weight work at the gym.

But recently, Keith had begun to complain about feeling tired all the time. An analysis of his nutrition and sleep habits revealed nothing unusual. At first, his physician thought his problem might simply be that he was wearing himself out by exercising too much.

Finally, however, after a complete physical exam, his physician was able to pinpoint the real problem: Keith was suffering from a low-grade sinus infection—apparently a recurrent condition that had been plaguing him off and on for years. Typical symptoms of this condition, all of which were experienced by Keith, include a chronic nasal drip, occasional low fevers that may escape detection, a general sense of fatigue, and an increased incidence of assorted aches and pains.

With the problem now identified, Keith's doctor knew that the condition called for a round of antibiotics. The medications knocked out the infection within two weeks and returned Keith to his normal, peppy self.

In this case, Keith employed an effective targeting strategy: he recognized that something was wrong with him physically, and he did an initial self-evaluation by pinpointing his particular symptoms and complaints. Finding that he was incapable of alleviating the problem on his own—and suspecting quite correctly there might be some underlying health condition—he turned immediately to his physician for help.

Unfortunately, many other patients with a sinus infection aren't aggressive enough to report their malaise to their doctors. Not only that, even when they do schedule an exam, the doctor sometimes misdiagnoses the sinus problem. At least once a month, I discover a patient with a low-grade sinus infection that is robbing him of his usual energy and zest.

The power of youth, then, often depends on something as simple as an alert patient who isn't afraid to report a loss of energy to his doctor—as well as on a doctor who is sharp enough to discern the correct source of the complaint.

CAUSE 2: FEELINGS THAT YOU ARE NO LONGER COMPETING AT YOUR PEAK

Those approaching age fifty and the years beyond may also suffer from youth drain—including a sense of being burned out—as they become tired of competing for promotions, or find their job skills are no longer fully appreciated. These feelings of career inadequacy are a primary source of many physical and emotional problems in a high percentage of my male patients who are among the four million baby boomers who have already turned fifty.

One of these men, "Tom," a fifty-two-year-old corporate marketing and public relations vice president, had always performed in the superior category on our standard treadmill stress test, which measures aerobic capacity and cardiovascular power. But in two consecutive medical exams, his stress test performances declined significantly. Even more ominously, he began to complain of chronic fatigue and a frequent aching sensation in his left arm.

These symptoms usually alert a physician to the possibility of some underlying disease, such as a heart problem, a malignancy, or a glandular disturbance. But after testing Tom for every likely physical cause of his problem, we found nothing.

So I began to question him about factors in his life that might be contributing to his problems. Soon I found the answer. Tom was confronting a major crisis at work: he was now the oldest person in his office, and it was clear that he would receive no further promotions, and probably no additional pay raises. Not only that, Tom's workload seemed to have increased, with extra demands to learn advanced computer technology, including special spreadsheet applications.

"I'm getting too old for this kind of stuff," he complained.

Gradually, the feelings of personal inadequacy and fears that he wouldn't be able to meet the expectations of his boss began to take their toll on him, both emotionally and physically. He found he was spending less and less time focusing on his family and his church and more and more time obsessing about his occupational problems. Also, he had put on hold a plan he had begun to develop to set up his own public relations business.

Fortunately, the symptoms Tom was experiencing hadn't yet reached the stage where he had developed a serious illness. But I knew if we failed to act soon, the worry and stress he was experiencing could easily result in high blood pressure, heart problems, or some other serious physical condition.

The Harvard School of Public Health conducted a twenty-year study, published in 1997 in *Circulation*, on the impact of worry among 1,759 older men. These men began without initial coronary heart disease. But by the end of the study, there were 323 cases of coronary heart disease, including 86 fatalities. The researchers concluded that high levels of worry—especially about one's social condition, self-definition, aging, finances, and health—may increase the risk of coronary heart disease in older men. (Vol. 95, pp. 818–24.)

To avoid such serious cardiovascular consequences, Tom had to take steps to eliminate from his life the constant, oppressive worries about being "past his prime" and "less competitive." This meant, first of all, achieving what the Harvard researchers in the above-mentioned study had called "self-definition"—a process which, for Tom, meant redefining his fundamental goals and values in life. Instead of focusing almost exclusively on his dead-end job and being tormented by the frustrations and anxieties surrounding it, he accepted the fact that he would never achieve any further promotions or pay raises in this particular company.

Of course, it wasn't enough for him simply to say, "I know I've reached the end of the line with this company"—and then to experience a near-magical transformation in his aspirations and expectations. Rather, Tom's achievement of self-definition required a multiphased effort, which began with a series of intensive reflections over a period of about a week on what his priorities in life should be.

Among other things, he resurrected the idea of starting his own PR firm. To this end, he began to plan ways he could start a viable sideline business—one that would give him some security in case he should lose his present job and also provide him with continuity in income when he finally did retire. Perhaps even more important, Tom began to devote more time to his family and church activities. During his time of reflection, he became profoundly aware of how his focus on work had almost pushed these important values out of the picture.

Tom's fundamental shift in his basic emphases in life helped eliminate his tendency to worry about his work. In effect, he began to develop a new identity with an enhanced sense of self-esteem. Soon, his chronic fatigue and the numbness in his left arm disappeared— and he reduced his risk of serious illness, including coronary heart disease. In short, Tom regained much of the personal energy, sense of excitement, and power of youth that he had lost because of a dead-end job.

CAUSE 3: TENSIONS CAUSED BY TIME PRESSURES

The primary slogan of our society could be, "So much to do, so little time." The pervasive sense of time pressure is potentially one of the most destructive of all the youth drains that rob us of our personal energy and vigor.

The time issue is evident in various surveys of the workplace, studies of leisure activities, and reports of the negative impact deadlines and crammed schedules have on human health. Consider, for instance, a study on work-home time interaction, which was released on April 15, 1998, in New York City by the Families and Work

Institute. The Institute found that work overload often starts a destructive office-home-office loop, which can cause ongoing stress and fatigue. The occupational time pressures typically build up on a given day and then spill over to damage the quality of home life.

Finally, the loop is completed when the worker returns to the office the following day. He may be overly tired because of excessive stress or preoccupied with guilt because of a failure on the previous evening to relate well to children and spouse. The end result is often an even lower capacity to function effectively on the job.

In this same vein, a survey by *Prevention* magazine (March 6, 1995) found that two-thirds of Americans say they feel stressed out at least once a week—and the health fallout from this stress, which is often time-related, can be devastating. For example, one hospital study of 791 patients at Beth Israel Deaconess Medical Center at Harvard University, published in March 1998 in *Circulation,* focused on "heart stoppers," stressful experiences that lead to heart attacks. The researchers found that those exposed to high-pressure deadlines within the seven days preceding their attacks faced 2.3 times the risk of heart attack as those without such deadlines. In other words, specific time pressures can lead to the ultimate youth drain: early death.

Time pressures may also trigger other health crises, such as poor nutrition and obesity in some people. In a preliminary study reported in March 1998, Yale researchers identified time constraints as a major cause of overeating. Appearing before a meeting of the Society of Behavioral Medicine in New Orleans, these scientists said that they had examined in depth the eating habits of sixty women, ages thirty to forty-five. They found that those under stress who had secreted the most cortisol—a potent steroid hormone put out by the adrenal gland—were also the ones who turned to high-fat foods to "treat" their stress. Such individual, biologically influenced responses will inevitably lead to a poor diet, excess body fat, and, therefore, a tendency toward chronic fatigue and other health problems.

Obviously, then, managing time pressures is one of the keys to regaining the power of youth—but how can you accomplish this feat?

Throughout this book, we'll be discussing various proven ways to respond to time demands—including new information on the role of exercise as an antidote to stress. But for now, just keep in mind the wisdom that has been passed on to us by Sarah Knauss, a one-hundred-eighteen-year-old Pennsylvanian who is currently the "oldest living woman," according to the *Guinness Book of Records*.

Born on September 24, 1880, in a small mining town, Mrs. Knauss has been in a nursing home since 1991. But she still manages to keep her mind active by following the course of current events in her daily newspaper. Also, she continues to enjoy her favorite foods—milk chocolate turtles, cashews, and potato chips—even though they might not pass muster by a Cooper Clinic dietitian.

But her main secret of a long life, as disclosed by her ninety-three-year-old daughter, Kathryn, deserves special kudos as a counter to the youth drain of time pressure: Mrs. Knauss is known as an "exceptionally tranquil person, and nothing fazes her."

This internal mastery over outside factors that tend to trigger tension and stress, such as time pressure, has long been recognized as a powerful protection against stress-related illness. Such illnesses, including heart disease and cancer, can destroy the power of youth and lead to untimely death.

Clearly, Mrs. Knauss has found a solution to this challenge. She has developed a remarkable inner balance, which has given her a mastery over those external time demands that are a major trigger of debilitating stress. (From an Associated Press report, April 19, 1998.)

CAUSE 4: THE PUNISHING EMOTIONAL AND PHYSICAL EFFECTS OF EXCESSIVE TRAVEL, INCLUDING BUSINESS TRAVEL

One of the most underestimated sources of youth drain is excessive travel. I ought to know, since I'm on the road nationally and internationally nearly six months out of every year. While journeying to give countless speeches, engage in business negotiations, or participate in medical presentations, I've logged millions of miles in airplanes, trains, and seagoing vessels. This travel has taken its toll in the form of cramped muscles, stiff joints, jet lag, and a variety of travel-related illnesses. When it gets out of control, travel can be one of the most destructive drains on emotional and physical health.

To counter the dangers of excessive business travel—and avoid the youth drain associated with them—a number of powerful preventive targeting techniques are available. Here's how these techniques can work:

First, you should identify the main dangers to health that are often associated with your business travel. Then, you're ready for the second step: apply specific responses to overcome those dangers.

More specifically, medical literature and the practical experience of many Cooper Clinic patients reveal these common danger areas with travel:

- jet lag
- diarrhea, fevers, and various infectious diseases
- sexually transmitted diseases
- road accidents
- skin cancers
- emotional ills, including depression and homesickness

The results of any of these health problems may range from the temporarily debilitating, to the potentially fatal. Yet just becoming aware of the dangers—and taking some simple, preventive precautions—can often greatly reduce the risks.

Take jet lag, for example, a problem suffered by almost every traveler who journeys between different time zones. Medically speaking, jet lag is the tendency of the body's circadian rhythm (inner time clock) to become desynchronized when you travel from one time zone to another. A number of negative physiologic responses may occur with jet lag, including disturbance of:

- sleep-wake patterns
- rhythms of catecholamines (bodily chemicals associated with stress, including adrenal hormones such as epinephrine)

- secretion of certain corticosteroids (steroids produced by the adrenal cortex)
- production of the hormone melatonin by the pineal gland
- overall mental and physical performance

Sometimes, after taking a series of back-to-back international trips, the effects are so debilitating that I begin to wonder if the normal inner rhythm and balance of my body have become permanently upset! Yet over the years, I've discovered a number of effective, medically proven responses to this problem. These responses can bring me back to normal within a day or two.

In the first place, aerobic exercise—including anything from light walking to a more demanding endurance workout—performed immediately after arrival in the new location is one powerful self-treatment that works for me. Furthermore, there is solid scientific support for my personal response.

In a 1996 Japanese study done at Yamaguchi University, researchers studied the effects of jet lag on airline crew members who flew from Tokyo to Los Angeles. Five crew members, averaging about forty-seven years of age, exercised outdoors for about five hours the day following their arrival in Los Angeles. Another five, a control group of the same age, stayed in their rooms and then went shopping after the flight.

The researchers found that both groups had similar hormonal and sleep-wake disturbances on the day of their arrival in Los Angeles, but they showed markedly different responses in their recovery from jet lag. The internal clocks and secretions of the exercisers became completely regularized—i.e., their jet lag was "cured"—on the day following their exercise. In contrast, the participants who did not exercise continued to suffer jet lag on that particular day.

The researchers concluded that outdoor exercise has an effect on hastening resynchronization of the inner biological clock when a person shifts to a radically different time zone. (See *Aviation and Space Environmental Medicine*, Dec. 1996; 67[12]: pp. 1155–60.)

Another specific response to jet lag that has worked for many people involves avoidance of caffeine and alcohol before sleep in the new location. Also, restricting sleep to the night hours, rather than trying to "catch up" on sleep during the day, can minimize jet lag. (See *Chronobiology International*, 1997; 14[2]: pp. 133–43.)

Certain drugs have also worked for some people, including hypnotic or sleep-inducing medications and melatonin. For example, studies have shown that melatonin has "chronobiotic" properties in humans, in that it is able to induce changes in inner biological rhythms, such as the body's core temperature and the sleep-wake cycle. But any such medications, whether prescription or over-the-counter, should be taken only under the supervision of a qualified physician. (See *Journal of Biological Rhythms*, Dec. 1997; 12[6]: pp. 604–17.)

On the other hand, there is no support at this point for the use of such "treatments" or blood thinner medications like heparin as bright lights to shift the sleep-wake cycle. (See *Thrombosis Research*, July 1996; 83[2]: pp. 153–60; *Chronobiology International*, March 1997; 14[2]: pp. 173–83.)

In addition to jet lag, there are many other challenges to health and well-being during travel, such as sexually transmitted diseases (STDs). In fact, STDs are the infectious conditions most commonly reported to health officials throughout the world. Some—herpes, for example—can cause serious permanent health problems. Others—specifically AIDS—can threaten life itself. (See *International Journal for the Study of AIDS*, Nov.–Dec. 1996; 7[7]: pp. 455–65.)

Some efforts have also been made to identify the types of travelers who pose the greatest risk of having or transmitting sexual diseases. In a 1997 Swedish report from Uppsala University, researchers studied 996 women, 276 of whom admitted that they had experienced casual sex during travel. Interviews with the women focused on their educational levels, sexual partnerships, reproductive history, contraceptive and drug use, smoking habits, and psychosocial factors such as wariness, success, and attractiveness.

The researchers determined that the women who were most likely to have had casual sex when traveling were single, had experienced broken relationships, were smokers, and were users of alcohol or marijuana. Also, their educational levels tended to be higher than those of women who avoided casual sex, and they were more likely to have a history of induced abortions. (See *Sexually Transmitted Diseases*, Aug. 1997; 24[7]: pp. 418–21.)

Other common travel diseases, which may undercut health and the power of youth, include dengue fever, especially among visitors to South America and Southeast Asia; diarrhea (the incidence varies from 8 percent to 50 percent of travelers, depending on the location); malaria; parasitic attacks; and skin infections. Skin infections, by the way, are among the six most frequent medical problems encountered by international travelers. (See *American Journal of Medicine*, Nov. 1996; 101[5]: pp. 516–20; *British Journal of General Practice*, Feb. 1997; 47 [415]: pp. 68–9; *Journal of the American Medical Association*, Dec. 3, 1997; 278[21]: pp. 1767–71; *Dermatological Clinics*, April 1997; 15[2]: pp. 285–93.)

The best way to guard against these diseases and infections while on the road is to first ask your physician about the specific health threats that you are likely to encounter on your trip. Then your doctor can help you prepare.

For example, he may provide you with medications, such as antibiotics that can be used to counter infections. Or he may simply remind you of important preventive practices in certain areas and countries, such as drinking bottled beverages and avoiding foods like lettuce and other fresh vegetables, which are likely to have been exposed to fecal matter or other contaminants.

The prospect of health threats from food while on the road is by no means limited to foreign travel, by the way. A recent study done by *The New York Times* of street vendors' offerings in New York City revealed that much of the food evaluated was undercooked, handled with unwashed hands, and subjected to unsanitary conditions. These factors raise significantly the risk of being infected by E. coli, salmonella, and other bacteria. (See May 17, 1998, p. 1.)

The best advice for people traveling is to do some research to find out which foods may pose the greatest risk. (A savvy physician can be of great help here.) Also, in general, stick to bottled drinks, well-cooked foods, and restaurants that have the reputation for being safe for travelers—and avoid unregulated snack stands, no matter how exotic they may appear.

Cause 5: Financial Worries

Another important cause of youth drain is ongoing anxiety about financial matters. I know from my own experience with near-bankruptcy a few years ago that when your livelihood is threatened, every ounce of your personal energy and vigor can be sapped by these concerns. (See *Can Stress Heal?*, pp. 169ff.)

Furthermore, the more serious the financial challenge you face, the more likely it is that you'll be emotionally and physically debilitated. In a 1997 article in the *New England Journal of Medicine*, researchers noted first that the relationship between a lower income and poor health is well established by scientific evidence.

Next, they reported on a study they had done among adults in Alameda County, California, who were facing economic hardship. The investigators found significant associations between those in hardship circumstances and all measures of their daily functioning. Specifically, they discovered that income problems impair such activities as cooking, shopping, walking, eating, dressing, and using the toilet. Also, those facing hardship are much more likely to suffer from clinical depression. (See Dec. 25, 1997, Vol. 337, No. 26, pp. 1889–95.)

What can you do to overcome your financial worries?

The best targeting response I know is to cultivate your spiritual life. Obviously, you should do all you can to earn an adequate living and manage your money wisely. But most of us at one time or another reach a point where our own resources are exhausted. An unanticipated home repair or a sudden illness may cause your money to run out before the next paycheck. You may even face the loss of a job at some time in your life. Situations like these are largely out of your control.

In such circumstances, the most powerful responses are spiritual. You've heard such sayings as:

- Let go and let God.
- Don't try to control the uncontrollable.
- Find the peace that passes understanding.
- Put your priorities in order: God first, family second, work third.

For more specifics on such "spiritual energy packs," see the discussion in Chapter 5 on "Hidden Energy Source #4: Advanced Spiritual Disciplines."

Unchecked worry is not only a youth drain, but it gives validity to another familiar saying: "You're going to worry yourself to death," as the next box explains.

Rx Response
Is Worrying Bad for Your Heart?

Researchers have often made a distinction between anxiety and worry. Specifically, anxiety refers to feelings—such as apprehension, fear, dread, restlessness, or tension—which may result from outside stresses, such as financial hardship. Worry is a response or coping mechanism to deal with this anxiety. For example, worrying may involve turning a particular source of anxiety over and over in your mind.

Sometimes, worry can be constructive, in that it can lead to solutions to the problem you are facing. But when no solution comes to mind, worry about personal finances can have a decidedly negative effect, including a harmful effect on your heart, according to a 1997 report from researchers at the Harvard School of Public Health. (See Laura D. Kubzansky, et al., "Is Worrying Bad for Your Heart?" *Circulation*, 1997; 95: pp. 818–24.)

CAUSE 6: UNEXPECTED EFFECTS OF MENOPAUSE—
BOTH MALE AND FEMALE

When someone mentions the loss of vigor with aging, one of the first things that comes to mind is sexual vigor. And there's absolutely no doubt that for both men and women, aging ushers in significant hormonal changes, usually accompanied by a decline in sexual functioning and desire.

For women, this change is commonly associated with menopause—the "change of life" that about twenty-five million females around age fifty undergo each year around the world. Hormonal shifts begin to occur, and these shifts radically alter the female sexual and reproductive capacities.

In particular, the internal production of the female hormone estrogen declines dramatically; the menstrual cycle halts; and the ability to reproduce ceases. As a result of these internal biological changes, menopausal women face an increased risk of such health problems as cardiovascular disease and osteoporosis. To counter these risks, they may go on hormone replacement therapy (HRT), which involves taking a combination of estrogen and progestin. (Caution: women with a history of breast or uterine cancer should not go on HRT. For other suggestions and caveats about HRT, see the discussion in Chapter 7.)

But the dramatic hormonal and sexual changes associated with aging are by no means limited to women. In fact, researchers have identified so many analogous transformations in men that some have taken to referring to a "male menopause," or "viropause." (See *Texas Medicine*, March 1997; 93[3]: pp. 53–5; *Clinical Geriatric Medicine*, Nov. 1997; 13[4]: pp. 685–95.)

In general, aging men experience a more gradual decline in their reproductive capacities than do women going through menopause. But there *is* a decline. For example, studies have established that there is a steady deterioration in semen quality in men over forty years of age—a change that is directly related to the aging process. (See *Archives of Andrology*, Nov.–Dec. 1995; 35[3]: pp. 219–24.) Also, aging apparently triggers a less efficient functioning of the male pituitary gland, which helps mediate testosterone levels. (See *European Journal of Endocrinology*, June 1995; 132[6]: pp. 663–7.)

Although there are significant differences between the male and female losses of sexual and reproductive vigor, there is no question about one thing: this time of life poses a number of serious, youth-draining dangers to members of both sexes. Here are some of the special challenges posed at this time of life—and a few suggestions about how targeting, in one form or another, may be able to help you respond to them.

Memory

Memory may become impaired after menopause—but estrogen can help bring it back. A 1997 Canadian study at McGill University in Montreal found that menopausal women who tended to have trouble with short-term and long-term memory could overcome their memory problems through estrogen treatments. The researchers concluded that estrogen helps maintain verbal memory and enhances the capacity for new learning in menopausal women. But other cognitive functions, such as visual memory, were apparently unaffected by the hormone. (See *Neurology*, May 1997; 48[5 Suppl. 7]: pp. S21–6.)

Libido

Libido does decline with age, but a high proportion of both men and women can remain sexually active in later life if they avoid the influence of myths and folklore. Researchers have determined that age-related physiological changes don't have to interfere with a meaningful sexual experience. In other words, there's no need for most people to succumb to the myth that as they age, they must regard themselves as "over the hill" sexually, or that they eventually will have to give up sexual relationships.

For example, studies have demonstrated that most men can continue to enjoy sex well into old age if they receive greater physical stimulation as part of sexual foreplay.

On the other hand, it's essential to be realistic. For one thing, both men and women will tend to enjoy sex more if they avoid the trap of expecting—or trying to force—the level of sexual response they enjoyed in their youth. For example, it's normal for most aging men to have more difficulty achieving or maintaining erections or not to experience orgasms with the same intensity that they did as teenagers. Also, women can expect to have less natural lubrication of their sex organs during intercourse. To compensate, they will have to rely on ointments, hormone therapy, or other medications prescribed by a gynecologist. (See *Western Journal of Medicine*, Oct. 1997; 167[4]: pp. 285–90.)

And remember: prescription medications designed to combat impotence, enhance orgasms, and promote ease of intercourse are becoming increasingly available. These include the impotence drug Viagra for men—which may also be helpful for women's orgasms, according to some preliminary findings. According to government estimates, thirty million men suffer impotence to some extent, often as a consequence of illnesses such as diabetes or medications such as those taken for hypertension. Preliminary reports suggest that Viagra and related medications may provide an effective response; however, some side effects have been reported. With Viagra, for instance, possible side effects include flushing of the face, headache, stuffy nose, mild decline in blood pressure, nausea, and a blue tint to vision.

Bone Mass and Muscle Strength

Both men over fifty and postmenopausal women tend to have problems with loss of bone mass and muscle strength, but weight-bearing exercise, including high-impact aerobics, can help both groups counter these threats.

In a 1996 British study at the Imperial College School of Medicine at St. Mary's, London, fifteen men and women, ages fifty to seventy-three, were assigned to do stepping and jumping exercises. These movements were designed to place a load on the proximal femur (uppermost part of the large leg bone that connects to the hip) and the spine. They exercised two to three times a week for one year, and then they were compared with a control group who did no exercise.

The exercise group experienced increased strength of their quadriceps (thigh muscles) and increased bone mass in their upper femur and hip bone. The researchers concluded that high-impact aerobic exercise in postmenopausal women and men over fifty can be effective in maintaining muscle strength and also in increasing the bone mineral density in the upper femur and hip bone. (See *European Journal of Applied Physiology*, 1996; 74[6]: pp. 511–7.)

Testosterone Supplementation

Testosterone supplementation therapy may be helpful in enabling some men to recover their sexual vigor after age fifty, but such therapy carries risks as well as potential benefits.

Many scientific studies have indicated that testosterone, the male sex hormone, has the power to improve bone mass and muscle mass in men older than fifty years of age. Also, this therapy may elevate the mood, improve the sexual functioning, and enhance the memory of some men.

But researchers caution that the long-term risks of this "androgen therapy" haven't been established yet, especially regarding its effect on cardiovascular disease and prostate cancer. (See *Journal of Andrology*, March–April 1997; 18[2]: pp. 103–6; *Clinical Geriatric Medicine,* Nov. 1997; 13[4]: pp. 685–95.)

I believe the safest approach is to avoid this type of therapy. The same goes for therapies employing melatonin, growth hormone, and DHEA (dehydroepiandrosterone), all of which have been recommended at some point for a more potent sex life. (For support of my position, see *Maryland Medical Journal*, April 1997; 46[4]: pp. 181–6.)

If for some reason you feel you must disregard this advice and explore the possibility of testosterone therapy—and you have found a qualified physician who recommends this approach—be sure that your physician first checks you thoroughly to determine your risk of cardiovascular disease and prostate problems. Also, he should continue to check your risk factors at least twice a year. In any event, you should be in the very low category of risk for both diseases before you even consider any therapy involving the administration of testosterone.

To sum up, then, I would suggest that you try other less risky responses to your virility problems before you go on a hormone regimen. One possibility is to consider making some changes in your lifestyle, which may slow the loss of this hormone.

In a 1997 study conducted by the Department of Epidemiology, Graduate School of Public Health, University of Pittsburgh, researchers examined the lifestyles, behavior, and testosterone levels of sixty-six men, ages forty-one to sixty-one, over a thirteen-year period.

They found that there were larger decreases in total testosterone among men who were heavy cigarette smokers and also those who were Type A personalities (tense and stress-prone). Also, the researchers found that decreases in the body's testosterone levels were associated with a rise in triglycerides (a blood fat) and a decrease in high-density lipoprotein (HDL, the "good" cholesterol that has been linked to a lower risk of heart disease). (See *American Journal of Epidemiology*, Oct. 15, 1997; 146[8]: pp. 609–17.)

Clearly, you should avoid smoking if you want to maintain higher levels of natural testosterone in your body. Also, effective stress management, especially for stress-prone Type A personalities, is a must.

Finally, there is a causal link between obesity and low HDL cholesterol, and there is likely a link between obesity and lower testosterone. I would suggest that men who want to regain the power of youth in their sex lives should lose excess weight and take steps to raise HDL levels. One proven way to raise HDL in many people is to engage in more aerobic (endurance) exercise, such as walking or jogging. So, does this mean that exercise will improve your sex life? Read on in the following box.

Can Exercise Increase Virility?

There has been a long-standing debate over what effect, if any, physical fitness and exercise can have on male sexuality. In other words, do bulging muscles, or tremendous aerobic power, automatically translate into sexual vigor?

The best answer to this question is, "No, but . . ."

That is, there is no clear causal connection between physical fitness and sexuality. Some highly conditioned athletes possess a relatively weak libido while plenty of couch potatoes have a high-powered sex drive.

But—and here is my all-important *but*—there is no doubt from our interviews with thousands of patients at the Cooper Clinic that physical fitness and conditioning, though no aphrodisiac, will improve your overall health, flexibility, endurance, and strength. As a by-product of these direct benefits, a sound exercise and nutrition program will most likely enhance the inherent sexual powers that have been bestowed on each person.

Beyond these rather generalized sexual benefits of fitness, some recent studies have identified hormone surges in both men and women who have engaged in exercise. In a 1996 study at the Division of Cardiology, University of Pittsburgh, researchers measured testosterone levels in seven sedentary but otherwise healthy men. These subjects, ages sixty-six to seventy-six, exercised for sixty continuous minutes on a stationary cycle. Blood samples were taken at ten-minute intervals for four hours before the exercise, during the workout, and for four hours following the exercise.

The researchers found that during the exercise, serum (blood) testosterone increased by 39 percent and a sex hormone-binding globulin by 19 percent. In the postexercise tests, hormone levels returned to normal.

The investigators noted in conclusion that short-term exercise has the ability to produce a transient elevation in blood testosterone levels in elderly men. (See *Metabolism*, Aug. 1996; 45[8]: pp. 935–9.)

Hormone changes were also noted in men and women after heavy-resistance exercise in a 1995 Finnish study. The researchers evaluated eight young women and eight young men in their thirties; seven middle-aged women and eight middle-aged men in their fifties; and eight elderly men in their seventies.

The participants were instructed to perform a heavy-resistance exercise program, with bench presses, sit-ups, and a bilateral leg press. Several sets of each exercise were done with the heaviest load possible. The recovery time between the sets was three minutes.

The scientists found that the mean concentrations of blood testosterone stayed the same for all the female groups. But significant increases in testosterone occurred in the young and middle-aged men. As for the elderly men, they showed no change at all in testosterone levels.

Measurements of levels of growth hormone—which is sometimes suggested as therapy for a loss of sexual vitality with aging—showed an increase in the young men and women and the middle-aged men and women. But again, the older participants showed no change in growth hormone levels as a result of the heavy exercise.

The researchers concluded that although younger people may be affected by a heavy-resistance workout, such exercise has little effect on sex or growth hormones in older people. (See *International Journal of Sports Medicine*, Nov. 1995; 16[8]: pp. 507–13.)

CAUSE 7: FRUSTRATIONS WITH CHILD REARING

Another important cause of youth drain involves the pressures, stresses, and strains related to child rearing.

Certainly, all of us who are parents know the joy of seeing a son or daughter negotiate the various stages of childhood, make it successfully to adulthood, and launch a satisfying career or marriage relationship. But along the way, we also know there are tremendous anxieties and stresses on Mom and Dad—any of which can rob us of the vim and vigor of youth.

The problem faced by many modern parents is summed up in a

1996 study conducted at the Department of Human Development and Family Life, University of Kansas. (See the *Journal of Pediatric Psychology*, June 1996; 21[3]: pp. 433–46.) The researchers there surveyed 413 parents of infants and toddlers about their child-rearing difficulties, behavior problems, and the parents' own need for support. Despite a high education and income level, the parents agreed on the whole that raising young children was a hard job. Their main difficulties focused on irritating behavior by the children, such as whining, refusal to obey parental requests, and interruption of adult activities. The parents who had more than one child and who had children two years old or older experienced the biggest problems.

Other sources of parental stress—and causes of youth drain—in child rearing include the following concerns.

The Impact of TV and the Mass Media

Many parents worry constantly about what TV programs or movies their children should view, how long they should watch, and what the short- and long-term impact of this entertainment may be on the youthful psyches.

Some recent studies and observations suggest there may be reason for concern. A study conducted at Stanford University and reported to the American Psychiatric Association's 1995 conference in Miami Beach revealed a disturbing impact of TV crime coverage on the emotions of children.

The researchers—who examined the national coverage of a 1993 kidnapping and murder of a twelve-year-old California girl—found that about 80 percent of 959 children interviewed were still thinking or dreaming about the crime two months after it was reported. The scientists concluded that children may be deeply affected emotionally just by being exposed to the news reports of a traumatic event.

An even more dramatic illustration of the impact TV can have on kids occurred in 1997 in Tokyo. A television network decided to cancel broadcasts of an action cartoon show because nearly six hundred child viewers, plus more than one hundred adults, were rushed to hospitals with convulsions, spasms, or nausea. Medical experts blamed the response on brilliantly flashing scenes in the program, which was typically viewed in small, crowded rooms.

Safety

Even though we live in a supposedly "civilized" society, the world where our children are growing up is full of traps and dangers. The very presence of these threats can exacerbate the normal anxieties and frustrations of child rearing.

For example, when teenagers become old enough to get driver's licenses and get out on the road by themselves, they and their parents automatically confront a frightening set of statistics. Even though the death rate among all drivers in the United States has declined over the past twenty years, the rate has nearly doubled for sixteen year olds. (See a 1996 study by the Insurance Institute for Highway Safety.)

Disintegration of the Two-Parent Family

Anxiety and preoccupation with troubled relationships—including the lives of children enmeshed in those relationships—are another source of much of the fatigue- and stress-related health problems I see at the Cooper Clinic.

Surveys and statistics concerning the American family reflect these destructive forces, which are ripping apart our family life. For example, since 1960, the percentage of families headed by single parents has more than tripled. In fact, single parents now head 30 percent of American families, according to reports from the U.S. Census Bureau.

The divorce rate, another barometer of family stability and health, has more than doubled since 1960. Half of all marriages now end in divorce, and many remarriages are breaking up as well. We have now reached the point where researchers estimate that 15 percent of all children in divorced families will see their closest parent remarry and then divorce again before the child turns eighteen. (See *The New York Times*, March 19, 1995, p. 1.) In the course of this process, about 30 percent of all children are now likely to spend some time in a stepfamily. (See *Demography*, Aug. 1995; 32[3]: pp. 425–36.)

As a result of these negative forces that are tearing apart our families, parents are faced with an increasingly heavy burden of having to deal with their kids' fears and other emotional problems. A Barna Research study has revealed that 65 percent of American children fear their parents might die; 53 percent fear poverty; and 51 percent fear they themselves may die.

Another 50 percent of our children fear kidnapping; 47 percent think their parents may not be "available" for them; 47 percent think they'll be unhappy in the future; and 45 percent are afraid of physical or sexual abuse. Predictably, 38 percent fear their parents will get a divorce at some point. (From a 1995 Barna Research poll, which surveyed 1,023 children for the KidsPeace organization.)

Don't assume, by the way, that this particular family-related youth drain is limited to the United States. An international survey, conducted in 1995 by the Population Council, a nonprofit group based in New York City, reported that in many developed countries, divorce rates doubled between 1970 and 1990. Also, unwed motherhood is exploding, with as many as a third of all births in Northern Europe occurring out of wedlock. (See *The New York Times*, May 30, 1995, p. A5.)

Clearly, the more problems a parent experiences personally, the more difficulties he will have bringing up a child successfully—and the more likely he'll begin to feel "old before his time." So what solutions, if any, are available to counter these stresses of child rearing?

Any suggestion for an easy targeting solution to these challenges must be discarded as simplistic. Instead, the best response seems to be to first accept the fact that there will inevitably be serious concerns and worries associated with raising a child. Then, having recognized the basic problem, do your best to strengthen your position as parents by working hard at building a strong marriage. Unfortunately, however, there are many cultural forces that are working against the development of solid marital relationships.

A common problem I've noted among many of my younger patients in the thirty to forty-five age range is that their marriage has been placed under unusual pressure because both spouses work. The stresses escalate exponentially if the working couple are simultaneously trying hard to bring up well-adjusted children.

One professional couple—I'll call them "Mark" and "Nikki"—present a typical picture. Both held down high-powered jobs that required them to be at work from early in the morning until early in the evening. As a result, on a typical day neither parent made it home before seven or eight at night. During the workday, their two children, ages five and nine, were either at school or under the care of a housekeeper.

When the entire family was finally together at night, it was almost time for the younger child to go to bed, and the older one followed in about an hour or so. This meant that Nikki and Mark were able to spend only about two to three hours a day during the week with both their children—a situation that produced an almost unbearable sense of frustration and guilt.

Stress levels in both spouses built up, with Mark developing marginally high blood pressure and Nikki experiencing chronic lower back problems. Both also complained of ongoing fatigue, a lack of interest in sex, and a sense of frustration: "Life is not satisfying for us right now because we don't have enough time for our kids or our own relationship."

The solution suggested for their nagging physical and emotional problems was to reduce stress levels by cutting back on their workload.

"After all," they were told, "you say that your children and your relationship with one another are your top priorities. Why not act on this conviction?"

But because they had come to rely on their joint income, neither could accept working fewer hours as a solution to their problems. They faced a kind of catch-22: their health, family life, and joy of youth were in jeopardy because of excessive work habits; yet they felt those very work habits were essential to support a truly happy and satisfying family life.

The case of Mark and Nikki provides a useful illustration of some of the findings of the 1995 Population Council study cited previously.

The other findings show that most of the changes occurring in families worldwide are directly linked to the increasing numbers of families with two working spouses.

The researchers noted that women actually work more hours each day than men, both at home and on the job. In twelve industrialized countries, employed women worked about 20 percent longer than employed men. In data from seventeen less developed countries, the situation was even worse: women worked 30 percent longer hours than men.

Such trends lead to more marriage breakups, less time for child rearing, more frustrations and anxieties, and acceleration of the aging process, especially for the wife. Because families have come to depend so heavily on both spouses' wages, the only reasonable solution to lessen the pressure on the woman—who typically puts in more hours on the job and at home—seems to be for the man in the family to take on more responsibility. (See the accompanying box on this subject.)

Pick-Me-Up
What Are Men Willing to Do Around the Home?

The 1991 National Survey of Men, published in 1996 in *Family Planning Perspectives*, revealed that 88 percent of the men interviewed strongly agree that a man has the same responsibilities as a woman for raising the children they have together.

On other family issues, a majority of the men (61 percent) believed that there is gender equality in sexual decision making, and more than three-quarters (78 percent) believe that men and women share equal responsibilities for decisions about contraception. (See *Family Planning Perspectives*, Sept.–Oct. 1996; 28[5]: pp. 221–6.)

So, there seems to be a basic willingness among men to participate with women in child rearing—and by implication, to take some of the time pressure off women around the home. Still, the question remains as to exactly how this sharing of the homemaking burden is going to work in practice. Other parts of the national survey indicate that men assume that women will typically take the lead role in making decisions about relationship issues, including sex. For most families, then, the answer may be for the woman to take the initiative in "assigning" the man various child-rearing tasks.

Clearly, there are no easy solutions to the age-hastening challenges of child rearing. But it's imperative for every mother and father to recognize the problem—and take whatever steps are necessary to reduce the stress levels associated with parenting.

Furthermore, a major concern isn't just the impact of your frustrations on you and your spouse—though those may be considerable and may rob you of the power of youth. Rather, the biggest problem is what neglect and stress in the family and in your marriage may do to your children.

Researchers at the 1998 annual meeting of the American Association for the Advancement of Science, held in Philadelphia, warned that babies may actually experience physical changes in their brains as a result of stresses they encounter during infancy. Among other things, scientists have discovered high levels of the stress hormone cortisol in crying babies.

What can be done to reduce the stress on infants in high-pressure modern-day households?

For one thing, busy parents, both male and female, can take more time to show a little tender loving care. Harvard investigators at the Philadelphia meeting said that infants who are forced to sleep alone or who are not picked up and comforted may develop post-traumatic stress disorder. The end result as adults may be a variety of health problems, including mental illnesses of various types. In short, the stresses that your children are experiencing right now may put them on a track to lose the power of youth by the time they barely reach adulthood.

CAUSE 8: EXHAUSTION FROM TECHNOLOGY AND INFORMATION OVERLOAD

In its May 5, 1997, issue, *The Wall Street Journal* ran a front-page story on executives in their fifties who had reached a ceiling on advancement and were having trouble adjusting to the new technology prevalent in today's business environment.

One fifty-four-year-old middle manager had learned to use a computer mouse within the past year and also had taught himself Microsoft Word and Excel. Even so, his younger colleagues made fun of his computer skills. The long hours required for learning new skills and at the same time finishing all his assigned work frequently left him exhausted at the end of his twelve-hour days.

Also, as one of the oldest people in his company—his boss was in his early forties—this manager reported that he felt frustrated because he knew he would never get another promotion at his present company. Yet, he had no prospects for moving on to another organization.

Others interviewed for the *Journal* article, who were in this manager's age range, expressed even more frustration at the acceleration of changes in their industries.

One fifty-year-old salesman said: "I just can't keep up. The products keep changing. The pressure to produce is relentless. To sell this last product, I had to learn more in a few weeks than I ever learned in college biology class."

Another fifty-four-year-old executive for a nonprofit organization that helps alcoholics and drug addicts said he would like a new job, but he complained, "I can't even understand most of the [want] ads. How many of those jobs could I respond to—maybe 5 percent?"

These responses are practical illustrations of what medical researchers have termed *technological stress* resulting from "psychophysiological symptoms" in modern offices. In one study done by the Department of Medicine, Karolinska Institute, Stockholm, Sweden, the investigators noted that increasing numbers of employees in modern office environments report psychosomatic symptoms.

They suggested that the reasons for the problems could be traced to high mental demands being made of those with a lack of sufficient skills. Also, they found that low organizational efficiency, as perceived by the workers, correlated with high mental stress. Many times, the researchers noted, the stress levels increased in offices as a result of "organizational reengineering." (This process may involve reorganization of the work environment, and sometimes the displacement of "unnecessary" workers, in an effort to increase efficiency.) Also, the investigators said, stress levels could soar with the introduction of new information technologies.

Those conducting this study concluded with the prediction that job-related psychosomatic problems will most likely increase in the foreseeable future because of the rapid changes that are occurring in the modern workplace. (See *Journal of Psychosomatic Research*, July 1997; 43[1]: pp. 35–42.)

CAUSE 9: WRONG EXPECTATIONS ABOUT YOUR HEALTH AND THE AGING PROCESS

Another pervasive cause of youth drain—which, in some respects, may be the most important—concerns inaccurate, and potentially dangerous, expectations. In other words, if you think you're getting old or past your peak, the chances are excellent that your low expectations about yourself will become a self-fulfilling prophecy.

A good illustration concerns a relatively young man by today's standards—a forty-nine year old who had always been a superb athlete and, in fact, had just won a singles tennis tournament at his athletic club. This man, whom I'll call "Lou," announced after his victory that because he was approaching fifty, he felt he was getting too old to subject himself to the strain of singles competition.

Apparently he had read somewhere that vigorous exercise at his age wouldn't do him any real good. In fact, he began to worry that challenging workouts might exert an unacceptable strain on his heart. So from now on, he said, he would concentrate on doubles—and would also cut back on his aerobic exercise sessions, which had involved jogging two to three miles twice a week.

When I heard about Lou's decision, I experienced a troubling wave of emotion—a mixture of frustration and anger. I was frustrated because I knew that Lou was in perfectly good health and that he had not been exercising excessively. In fact, given his relatively fit condition, he could easily have increased the amount of exercise he was doing with no ill effects. But by cutting back on his activity, he was sure to lose the edge provided by the conditioning he had achieved. The advantages that he had been enjoying included a high level of stamina and endurance in his daily life, a stable weight and percentage of body fat, as well as the statistical probability of living longer.

I was also angry about Lou's decision because he had been reading material by so-called "experts" with whom I've been debating for years. These pundits, some of whom are physicians, have made a career of trying to persuade the public that exercise isn't particularly important or healthy. Unfortunately, they have had some success in chipping away at the overwhelming scientific evidence that demonstrates clear health benefits of a moderate to high level of fitness.

One such piece of evidence is the landmark study conducted at the Cooper Institute for Aerobics Research and published in the *Journal of the American Medical Association* on November 3, 1989. That report has established that only thirty minutes of sustained activity, such as fast walking, three to four times each week will have a significant impact on reducing deaths from all causes. Furthermore, the researchers, led by Dr. Steven Blair of the Institute, found that doing a little more exercise, of the type that Lou had been used to, will statistically reduce even further a person's likelihood of dying prematurely from all causes.

In short, there was absolutely no reason for Lou to cut back on his regimen, and there is every reason for him to stay with it. But he had convinced himself that his "advancing age" made it wise for him to reduce his activity level, and no amount of arguing was going to change his mind.

There's also an interesting and encouraging final chapter to this story. When I heard from Lou a year after he had embarked on his new "age-adjusted" fitness regimen, he was not at all happy with the results. He had put on twelve pounds, was experiencing more aches and stiffness in his back and legs, and reported that he had begun to run out of steam far too early in the afternoon. In fact, many days he seemed to have no energy at all, and he found he couldn't even think clearly when he was presented with new problems at work.

Clearly, Lou's undemanding fitness program wasn't working well. His expectations about his health and the aging process had indeed become a self-fulfilling prophecy. Although at first he couldn't quite figure out why his sense of physical and emotional well-being had deteriorated, he soon realized what had happened. As soon as he did, he returned to the more vigorous fitness regimen that was appropriate for his not-so-advanced age. He also won his club's singles championship again the following year.

To sum up, then, Lou had discovered an essential principle about how to grow older happily and successfully: to a large extent, your mind and emotions determine how well you age. Consider a few real-life illustrations of how this power of positive expectations can work to provide a youth-booster effect:

Those who have retained the power of youth expect to retain their staying power at work. The most obvious example of this trait is the new Iron Man of baseball, Cal Ripken Jr., who in September 1995 surpassed Lou Gehrig's record for consecutive major league baseball games played—a phenomenal 2,131 games over more than thirteen seasons.

Shortly after Ripken's achievement, *The New York Times* (Sept. 17, 1995, p. 11) cataloged the exploits of some less well-known iron men and women. They included a number of people who had even more impressive consecutive-workday records than the baseball star:

- Bob Garland, a seventy-six year old who had worked nonstop in his milk business in Anson, Maine, from 1939 to 1992

- Grace Chewning, the fifty-eight-year-old city clerk of Orlando, Florida, who had not missed a day of work from 1960 to 1995
- Lore Noto, original producer of the record-running off-Broadway musical *The Fantasticks*, who had been involved in 6,438 straight performances, from 1970 to 1986, according to the *Guinness Book of World Records*
- The late U.S. Supreme Court Justice Potter Stewart, who had never missed a day in his twenty-three years on the Court

These people listed a number of possible sources for their impressive stamina on the job, including the excitement of competition, a special love of the job, and a strong sense of duty and responsibility. Perhaps most important of all, they all seemed to have retained the power of youth at work because they looked forward to the challenges that each new day brought into their lives.

Older people with the power of youth want to live longer. These people display an innate survival instinct—even if their health begins to decline.

Various diseases and health problems are inevitable as we age, but that doesn't mean that the mind-set of youthfulness must be lost. In fact, the *Journal of the American Medical Association* reported in its February 1998 issue that people in their eighties and nineties preferred to live longer, even if they had the choice of a shorter life in better health. In other words, these older patients had an innate drive to achieve an extended *quantity* of life, not just an improved *quality* of life.

This survival instinct—the drive to keep on going and living, no matter what the hardship—is a common characteristic of many of my patients, who often do prevail over difficult health problems.

Older people with the power of youth press to have new experiences, even if some may object they are too old. Perhaps because I used to do testing and training for NASA when I was in the air force, the most obvious examples of this principle that come to my mind are the intrepid band of older astronauts.

I'm reminded of Story Musgrave, the sixty-one-year-old space veteran who, on November 8, 1997, became the oldest human in space. And of course, there's Senator John Glenn, who, while in his late seventies, volunteered to go back into space to evaluate the effects of space and weightlessness on the aging process.

This attitude of always looking for a new adventure, a new frontier to conquer, will go a long way toward keeping the aging mind fresh and expectations high.

Older people with the power of youth refuse to let physical problems get them down. One of the most important qualities that enable older people to retain the power of youth—and fend off the effects of youth drain—is the ability to rise above physical setbacks and disabilities when they strike. I maintain an ongoing file of amazing people who have not only mastered their health problems, but have often gone well beyond those who are supposedly whole and healthy. Here is a sampling:

- A heart transplant recipient, Robert Skaretka, entered the New York City Marathon held on November 12, 1995. The forty-six-year-old Skaretka's feat was his fourth New York City Marathon since he got his new heart in April 1991. His approach is to walk quickly most of the way, though he does speed up to a run on occasion.
- A seventy-six-year-old Inverness, Florida, woman, Norma Wickwire, was listed in the *Guinness Book of Records* in 1998 as an example of "Medical Extremes." Called the "Bionic Grandma," she kept her spirits up by remaining as active as possible, even though doctors had replaced eight of her ten major joints—both hips, both knees, both shoulders, an ankle, and an elbow. Her children reported that she had refused to allow osteoporosis and rheumatoid arthritis, which had plagued her since 1968, to get her down.
- German-born Anneliese Monniere, who lost the use of her legs while she was in her fifties as a result of a bicycle accident, refused to succumb to this setback. She first learned to stand and then to walk around the house. Before long, she was walk-

ing outside and jogging on occasion. Two years after her accident, she entered her first marathon. In the ensuing decade or so, she ran in marathons in Africa, Russia, Bermuda, China, Germany, and the Himalayas. At last report, in the spring of 1998 at age seventy, she was still going strong, having entered a California run to raise money for the Leukemia Society of America.

Older people with the power of youth discipline themselves to put their inner lives in order. A study of centenarians done by Lynn Adler revealed that older people seem more spiritual than those who have not reached the hundred-year mark. In a survey of three thousand centenarians, she discovered that nearly all the respondents rated religion and spirituality among the most significant aspects of their lives. (See *The Wall Street Journal*, Dec. 31, 1997, p. 1.)

This same attitude is reflected in many of the case studies I've compiled over the years. For example, a one-hundred-four-year-old former hairdresser, Edmond Hontans, who lives in Hobe Sound, Florida, was a former bodybuilder. To keep in shape, he still lifts light weights during exercise sessions at his nursing home, even though he gets around by wheelchair.

When questioned about his secret for a long, active life, he acknowledged the importance of staying physically active and also noted that he never smoke or drank, except for an occasional glass of wine. But he said, "The best thing is to be a disciple of God. I'm privileged to be close to God." (See *The Palm Beach Post*, Oct. 7, 1997, p. B1.)

If I had to sum up my own response to these various treatments, I'd say that perhaps the best single antidote to youth drain is to nurture your inner life. In part, this means disciplining yourself to remain optimistic and upbeat about your prospects for enjoying good health and happiness as you grow older. This sort of "inner treatment" is by far the best treatment for those daily stresses that sap us of the energy and vigor we enjoyed to the full in our youth.

Of course, staying upbeat about aging is not so easy because gerontophobia, the fear of aging, can grip our minds and make us expect the worst about our future. On the other hand, a solid dose of reality can be good medicine for this sort of pessimistic fantasy.

Consider one recent study, which confirmed that people under age fifty tend to be pessimistic about aging. Yet the study also showed that the reality of aging is quite different: those who had already retired and were on Social Security believed that aging wasn't all that bad! (From a poll released on April 4, 1998, by the Americans Discuss Social Security Project.)

Here are some of the specific fantasies and realities identified by the study:

- *Fantasy*: 29 percent of those eighteen to forty-five years old expect to become dependent on their kids.
  Reality: only 8 percent of individuals over eighty say that has actually happened to them.
- *Fantasy*: about half of those surveyed under age fifty expect a serious illness to befall them when they are older.
  Reality: only 32 percent of those over eighty have actually encountered such an illness.

What important lesson can we draw from these findings?

It would seem that the reality of aging is that our later years are likely to be much more attractive than what our fears and expectations suggest. Furthermore, those who expect the worst are most likely going to start feeling more tired and unwell, while those who expect to retain their youthfulness will most likely hold on to the power of youth well into old age. So never underestimate the power that your mind has to affect your physical and emotional makeup, whether for evil or for good!

To sum up, then, when you are evaluating yourself on the Cooper Energy Scale introduced in Chapter 3, it should be helpful to begin with a checklist based on the five energy sappers described in that chapter, plus the nine causes of youth drain detailed in this chapter.

Here they are once again:

- general bad stress
- depression
- inadequate sleep
- a pessimistic attitude
- dehydration
- nagging, recurring health complaints
- feelings that you aren't competing at your peak
- tensions caused by time pressures
- excessive travel
- financial worries
- unexpected effects of menopause, male or female
- frustrations with child rearing
- exhaustion from technology or information overload
- wrong expectations about health and aging

If you're feeling old, tired, or otherwise out of sorts, the chances are that one or more of these fourteen factors are the source of your problem. In this case, you have a ready set of reminders here to help you make a quick evaluation of yourself on the Cooper Energy Scale.

But you may also find significant help with several other "hidden," or frequently overlooked, sources of personal energy. These secrets of stamina, which should be useful for anyone of any age, can provide you with even more power as you respond to the low-energy entries on your energy scale.

5
• • • • • • • • • • • • •

The Overlooked Secrets of Stamina— for Every Age

When low energy is a problem, high-profile solutions often get most of the press. These include a number of responses to fatigue that we've already begun to discuss, including targeted exercise routines, "nutrimedicine" (or specially prescribed nutritional responses), and achieving sound sleep.

But because these strategies are so obvious—and because they often provide such powerful antidotes when we're trying to overcome fatigue and regain youthful vigor—it's easy to overlook four other, lower-profile approaches, which may work just as well, or even better.

These "secret" sources of stamina include:

- stimulating personal creativity
- finding a peaceful place
- laughing
- developing advanced spiritual disciplines

So when you find you are registering too low on the Cooper Energy

Scale, first go through the checklist and various "targeting treatments" suggested in the previous chapters. But if you find you're still having problems with your personal energy levels, try one or more of the following additional targeting strategies, which may provide just the "hidden source" of youthful vigor that you need.

HIDDEN ENERGY SOURCE 1: PERSONAL CREATIVITY

The power of the mind over the body begins to approach a peak as we exercise our creative powers effectively. In other words, if you're tired, turn to some creative outlet, and watch your energy levels be transformed.

Reflect for a moment on how energized you have felt after:

- completing a new, groundbreaking project at work
- engaging in a conversation that helped another person change his life for the better
- spending your spare time on a project that helped someone less fortunate than yourself
- reading a book that stimulated you to think or act in new directions
- participating in an athletic event during which you entered a "zone" of super-high, effortless performance
- devoting a few hours to a satisfying artistic pursuit, such as painting, music, or writing in a journal

These and countless other possibilities illustrate the potential for creative expression. Almost inevitably, the emotional and spiritual aftermath of such experiences catapults us to a higher level of vigor and expectation about ourselves. Of course, a key ingredient of the power of youth is the recapturing of that exciting sense of passion and possibility about ourselves and the future that characterized us at one time or another when we were much younger.

How can you generate more creativity in your life?

Here are some suggestions that I have gleaned both from my most energetic patients and from experts I encounter in many fields, who never seem to run out of ideas or a sense of excitement:

Read as Much as Possible

Ideas generate creativity, and one of the best ways to get new ideas is to become widely read. You may think you don't have enough time to do extra reading. But before you give up, consider the example of Sir John Templeton, the founder of the Templeton group of mutual funds, and widely regarded as one of the premier investment experts of all time.

Templeton acknowledged a few years ago that he regularly worked at least sixty hours per week, half on his business and half on his religious and philanthropic projects. But he still found time to read extensively by being sure to carry a sheaf of articles and other materials with him when traveling around the world, or going to a business meeting.

Inevitably, during these "open spaces" between meetings and engagements, he would be able to read the latest reports on stocks that he was considering purchasing, or philosophical and theological discourses that helped him in his philanthropic decisions. (See William Proctor's *The Templeton Touch,* Doubleday, Garden City, NY, 1983, pp. 91–92.)

Of course, it's important to choose the reading materials that will help generate ideas. Potboiler novels may provide some relaxation, but they probably won't stimulate thinking in particular new or creative directions that may be most useful to you. For this reason, John Templeton has avoided novels altogether.

In my own case, I continue to do a new book every year or so because the required research into new areas of medicine and related topics helps maintain the flow of "creative juices" in my own life. In the last ten years, reading extra material on antioxidants, folic acid, stress, and longevity has helped me think in new directions, and has led to the authorship of several new books in these areas.

Pick-Me-Up
Can Exercise Really Enhance Creativity?

Researchers from the School of Psychology, Middlesex University, United Kingdom, noted in a 1997 report that scientific literature has established that various forms of physical exercise—even a single workout—can promote a positive mood. Also, they acknowledged that there was some evidence that physical exercise may enhance creative thinking.

For one thing, they said positive moods can provide a favorable context for creative thinking. Also, there is a large amount of anecdotal literature suggesting that creative people sometimes use bodily movement to help overcome "blocks" to their creative thinking.

But in this study, which appeared in September 1997 in the *British Journal of Sports Medicine* (Vol. 31, No. 3, pp. 240–5), the investigators focused more specifically on whether creative thinking after exercise was attributable to the improved mood fostered by the exercise.

They evaluated the responses of the sixty-three participants to exercise (an endurance exercise such as fast walking or aerobic dance) and to watching a video presentation. Mood was measured by asking the participants to assign an adjective to the way they felt, and creative thinking was tested with a standard measure known as the "Torrance test."

The results of the study revealed a significant increase in positive mood after exercise and a significant decrease in positive mood after the video presentation. After evaluating all the tests, the researchers concluded that both mood and creativity were improved by exercise, but that they were affected by the physical workout independently of one another. In other words, the improvement in creativity did not depend on the improvement in mood.

Take Reasonable Risks

As we grow older, the tendency is to settle into those activities and work assignments that are most familiar. Humans gravitate toward the familiar because the familiar is comfortable. Something deep inside often seems to whisper, "Choose immediate comfort, or what feels good for the moment. Avoid more challenging experiences that seem to have a more uncertain outcome."

Following this path—and failing to step out in an entirely new direction—is a sure way to boredom, burnout, and low energy levels. On the other hand, taking a chance on the unknown is often the quickest path to extraordinary insights and achievements, and the discovery of powerful new sources of personal vigor.

The only qualification I would suggest is that the risk you take be reasonable. Obviously, you don't want to sink your life savings into a wild, unsubstantiated idea, which you haven't explored with plenty of research. But if your research suggests that this venture is indeed rational and promising, then consider taking a plunge!

For example, take my experiences in breaking new ground in preventive medicine, which I have detailed in a number of other books, most notably my *Aerobics* and *Antioxidant Revoution.*

It was certainly a forbidding, uncomfortable prospect for me to challenge the Dallas medical establishment by advocating treadmill stress testing. Or to promote more exercise for the over-forty set when that was considered the time of life to slow down. Or to recommend antioxidant supplements when most doctors were opposed to the idea. Yet in each of these cases, the discomfort generated creative thinking, excitement—and increasing amounts of personal energy in my life.

Learn New Skills

Perhaps the most effective way to stymie your creative side is to become stalled in the acquisition of new skills. I highly recommend that, whenever possible, you take advantage of expanding your knowledge—especially your practical knowledge, which may launch a new avocation, or make you more efficient in your chosen vocation. Here are a few cases in point:

Music. I've known a number of people who either resurrected an old music skill that they had developed when they were quite young, such as piano lessons, or started from scratch when they were in their thirties, forties, or even older.

One attorney, for instance, decided to start taking piano lessons for the first time when he was in his early forties. This new skill opened up an entire array of other interests, such as listening to recorded classical music and attending concerts. Not only did he add an extra dose of passion to his after-work life, but the enthusiasm also spilled over into his work. He found a new sense of peace and positive thinking just by exposing himself regularly to good music.

Computers. Although an increasing number of older baby boomers are learning the ins and outs of computer use and the Internet, many are still "computer-phobic." I must say that I've been in this latter category until just recently. It's been too easy to allow my executive secretary and other assistants to do the hands-on computer work, and to avoid any personal interaction with the strange new technology. But an introduction to E-mail and to online medical research resources has begun to fascinate me—and I expect that I'll continue to expand my creative potential in this area.

Youth Booster
Can Computers Work Against Creativity?

Although computers and Internet "surfing" can certainly expand your knowledge and enhance creativity in many people, the technology may actually work against your creative impulses if you have "computer anxiety."

A study done at Buckinghamshire College in Great Britain and reported in April 1997 in *Psychology Reports* (Vol. 80, No. 2, pp. 395–402) explored the relationship of "cognitive spontaneity" to computer anxiety and attitudes toward computer use. The 178 subjects who were evaluated were attending advanced management courses.

The investigators found a significant negative relationship between computer anxiety and cognitive spontaneity—a freedom of thought that is a major ingredient of creativity. The negative impact of anxiety on creativity held up even when the researchers took into account the computer experience of the participants.

Those doing the study concluded that their results showed both a direct and indirect relationship between cognitive spontaneity and computer anxiety.

I recommend that if you are involved with computers but feel you are beset by computer phobia or anxiety, immerse yourself in a computer course or other intense learning experience. Knowledge and regular practical exposure to the fear are good remedies for anxiety.

Sports. Just because you've passed the milestones of fifty, sixty, or even seventy, don't assume that you can't learn new athletic skills! Of course, the older you are, the more important it is to ease into the new activity and to take pains to prepare yourself physically for strange movements. But age should not be a deterrent. Check some of the stories in the longevity discussion in Chapter 10, and you'll get a taste for what's possible, even at an advanced age.

Vary Your Daily Routine

Most people become bored by repetition—whether it's at work, at home, or on the playing field. Even those who claim to prefer a completely predictable life—such as going to the same restaurant every Friday night, eating the same food, and returning home at the same time—could benefit from a little variety.

One good example of the advantages of variety is evident in the design of an effective exercise routine. As you'll see in the following chapter, I'm a big believer in the concept of "cross-training," or mixing up an exercise regimen to include several different athletic activities. In other words, in my own regimen I include fast walking, jogging, cycling, mountain hiking, skiing, and strength training with resistance apparatuses. Obviously, I don't pursue all of these activities every week or even every month. But in a typical week, I will include at least three or four of them, and when I'm on vacation in Colorado, I may plug most of them into my workout.

There are several reasons for varying many aspects of your daily routine. One is that the more variety you experience, the less likelihood there is that you'll become bored and give up. Another reason is that the wider your experience, the more skills you'll develop—and the more likely it is that you'll protect yourself.

Cross-training in sports, for instance, helps develop supporting muscles that may prevent overuse problems and injury. A kind of "cross-training" at work—where you learn a variety of different skills—will provide potential fallback positions in case you lose your job: if you know computers as well as management skills, you'll be a step ahead of the person who only knows management.

Finally, injecting variety into your life will enhance your creativity. You may not automatically see how a new skill in music or computers or tennis will make you think more creatively on the job, or improve your problem-solving skills. But believe me, the more you open your mind to new concepts and learn to think in other contexts—or "out of the box" as some "creativity consultants" have called the process—the more effective you'll be in furthering your career or avocational objectives.

Seek Input from Others

Go out of your way to consult with others—and meet new people.

The birthplace of many new ideas is in brainstorming sessions. Obviously, you can't brainstorm by yourself; other people are necessary. So even if you are in a relatively solitary occupational setting, where you don't have to interact too much with other people, it's wise to seek out forums where you can toss new ideas back and forth.

Too often, even those who are exposed regularly to others don't listen or respond adequately to fresh ideas and suggestions. This is especially the case with high-level managers and executives, who are used to having others follow their orders and respect their opinions.

Because I'm the chief executive officer and the founder of the various operations I oversee—the Cooper Clinic, the Cooper Institute for Aerobics Research, and the Cooper Aerobics Center—I'm particularly vulnerable to the danger of making decisions in a vacuum, without adequate input from other experts. Fortunately, however, I'm surrounded by a group of professionals who are willing to "talk straight" to me—and I appreciate their honesty.

Sure, I can be thin-skinned, and criticism can be as painful to me as the next person. But whenever I find myself becoming defensive, I recall the words in Proverbs: "Without counsel, plans go awry, / But in the multitude of counselors they are established" (15:22 NKJV).

I've encountered many situations where one of my ideas, or a concept suggested by one of my colleagues, was quite creative and promising. But if we had proceeded on that basic idea without further input, we would have failed. On the other hand, when the original idea was shaped and refined by the suggestions and critique of others, we were in a much better position to succeed.

Here, we come to the importance of the second part of this principle: generating ideas by meeting and working with new people.

With many of my books and projects—such as the national bestseller *Controlling Cholesterol*, books on osteoporosis and hypertension, and the controlled production and testing of our recent vitamin offering, Cooper Complete—I've always relied heavily on the expert input and creativity of others. Such world-renowned medical experts as Dr. Scott Grundy, Dr. Charles Pak, Dr. Norman Kaplan, Dr. Jacob Selhub, and Dr. Walter Willett have added immeasurably to my own efforts.

Follow Sound Health Habits

This final suggestion for improving your capacity for creative thinking may seem almost too obvious to be mentioned. But unfortunately, it's often overlooked—with disastrous results.

The basic principle could be stated this way: you can't think straight at all, much less creatively, if you fail to get enough sleep, eat wisely, and get regular exercise.

When I find my own thinking processes stymied, and my creativity nonexistent, the first thing I do is examine my sleep: Am I getting the minimum six and a half to seven hours a night that I need, or have I slipped back into that old five to five and a half hours a night habit?

Then, I'll check my nutrition: Have I been eating on schedule, or am I allowing my packed scheduled to push my mealtimes back to an unusually late hour, or to push them out of the picture altogether?

Finally, I'll take a look at my exercise routine: Has my frenetic travel schedule caused me to skip too many workouts per week? If I'm feeling fatigued or fuzzy-headed, the chances are that I need to adjust my schedule so as to plug an adequate amount of aerobic and strength training back into my daily routine.

Creativity, then, is the first "secret source" of energy that you should always consider tapping into if you find you are turning in a low score on the Energy Scale. The second secret source is one that many people take years to discover, if they find it at all—finding a peaceful place.

HIDDEN ENERGY SOURCE 2: A PEACEFUL PLACE

In our high-voltage, success-oriented, competitive culture, it's almost impossible to get away from other people. We are advised about how to influence others to enhance our chances for success— for instance, conducting and participating in effective meetings, operating in "team" situations on the job, functioning well in personal relationships and family settings, and interacting productively with our children.

Unfortunately, we are told very little about how to be alone—even though a time of productive solitude can be one of the greatest resources of well-being and youthful power. In other contexts, I've discussed the importance of the personal "retreat" as an antidote to stress. But here, I'm talking about something more comprehensive and positive: finding a "peaceful place" is the secret to regrouping your energies, rethinking your priorities and relationships, and preparing to "fight another day" in the demanding world of daily relationships and work.

Here are a few suggestions that have proven effective, either for me or for my colleagues and patients:

Set Aside Time for Reflection

Try to start off every day with at least fifteen minutes to a half hour for some quiet evaluation of the upcoming work schedule or maybe prayer, devotions, or Bible reading—or all of the above. If you set a calm, measured tone at the beginning of the day, the rest of your schedule will be more likely to fall into line naturally, with a minimum of anxiety and stress. (This practice fits naturally into the "Spiritual Monitor" concept discussed later in this chapter.)

Set aside a time for solitary reflection at the end of the day also. This end-of-day ritual is designed to quiet your mind just before you go to sleep. The focus should not be on worries and pressures of the previous day or the one to come, but on peaceful thoughts. Reading one of the Psalms has often worked for me.

Design a Quieter Office Space

The senior design engineer at Steelcase, the nation's largest office-furniture maker, has said that the human voice is the most distracting sound in the office. On the other hand, complete silence can be as distracting as too much noise. For most people, the best solution in somewhere in the middle, with enough background noise to overcome complete silence, but not so much as to become distracting.

One way to deaden sounds, including extraneous conversation, to the desired level is the strategic use of acoustical panels. Steelcase and other furniture designers are constantly testing these for use both in regular offices and in cubicles, which are only closed in on the sides, not on the top.

So if you're having trouble finding a quiet space to work, don't just accept your current noise level as inevitable. Check your local office furniture outlet to see what solutions may be available. (See *The Wall Street Journal,* Aug. 21, 1995, p. B3.)

Try Gardening

Some people find their most effective "quiet place" when they're moving about, rather than sitting still. One of the most effective ways to achieve solitude and engage in a kind of soothing self-therapy while on your feet is gardening.

Fred Law Olmstead, one of the greatest landscape designers in American history, who designed Central Park in New York City, believed that plants have the power to employ the mind without causing fatigue. In this tradition, a number of organizations, such as the American Horticultural Therapy Association, have sprung up to promote emotional well-being through gardening.

We are at the very beginning of scientific research into this subject, but the first wave of findings is encouraging. For example, researchers at the University of Illinois at Champaign-Urbana have reported that crime rates fell among those living in a Chicago public housing project where trees had been planted. Also, efforts are being made to combine gardening with treatment and healing for patients with autism and other conditions.

I have a number of patients and friends who regularly turn to their gardens for peace and refuge from the stresses of daily life. Inevitably after they have emerged from one of these sessions, they report experiencing a surge of extra physical energy—and they actually look younger!

Come to think of it, maybe I should begin to raise orchids myself!

HIDDEN ENERGY SOURCE 3: LAUGHTER

The healing and energizing effects of laughter and good humor have long fascinated philosophers, physicians, and psychological counselors. As long ago as the seventeenth century in England, Robert Burton, Anglican clergyman and author of the classic *Anatomy of Melancholy,* said: "Humor purges the blood, making the body young and lively, and fit for any manner of employment." (See the essay in *Radiology Technology,* Sept. 1997; 69[1]: pp. 83–7.)

Contemporary therapists in a variety of settings acknowledge that a sense of humor and ability to laugh can be therapeutic for both the patient and the caregiver. A review article in *Dermatology Nursing* (Dec. 1997; 9[6]: pp. 423–9), for instance, reports that good humor and laughter can reduce stress, enhance hope, relieve tension, and stimulate the immune system.

Although most experts recognize that much of the evidence in this area is anecdotal, and that more extensive studies need to be conducted, many have sufficient confidence in the healing and energizing power of laughter to advocate the use of various types of "laughter" therapy. For example, at the Cancer Center, Presbyterian Hospital, Charlotte, North Carolina, caregivers have developed a "Laugh Mobile" to raise the spirits of hospital patients. This hall-roving vehicle includes displays of humorous novelties, books, and films, which are designed to divert the attention of the suffering patients to lighter thoughts. (See *Oncology Nursing Forum,* Nov. 1991; 18[8]: pp. 1359–63.)

Also, nurses and physicians have learned to look for the presence or absence of signs of good humor as a "behavior marker" for recovery in patients with major depression. Important markers include the social smile, raised eyebrows, wrinkled eyebrows, social laughter, gesticulation, and social interest. (See *Journal of Nervous Mental Disorders,* March 1998; 186[3]: pp. 133–40.)

Other uses of laughter and good humor in medical treatment include:

Increasing Pain Tolerance

Research has shown that humor has the power to distract patients from their discomforts and increase their pain tolerance.

It may be that the reason that laughter works is the release of endorphins (morphine-like neurotransmitters that produce a feeling of well-being) and the reduction of tension. Or it's possible that humor distracts the patient from his or her pain.

For example, in the November 1995 issue of *Pain* (Vol. 63, No. 2, pp. 207–12), researchers from Bar-Ilan University, Department of Psychology, Ramat-Gan, Israel, exposed four groups of pain patients, consisting of twenty subjects each, to four separate situations. These included watching a funny film, a repulsive film, a neutral film, or no film.

The results showed that both the humor and repulsive film groups enjoyed the greatest increase in pain tolerance.

Saving Suicidal Patients

Investigators at the Albert Einstein College of Medicine, Bronx, New York, have found that where laughter and humor are used during therapy with suicidal and depression patients, five principles emerge: 1) The freedom to be humorous is part of a positive doctor-patient relationship. 2) Humor is life-affirming. 3) Humor increases social cohesion. 4) Humor is interactive. 5) Humor reduces stress.

The researchers determined that the main effects of good humor are symptom relief and enhancement of relationships. They recommended that health practitioners make optimal use of humor in their treatments. (See *Gerontologist,* April 1995; 35[2]: pp. 271–3.)

Laughing Meditation

Some therapists have gone beyond simply trying to evoke spontaneous laughter in their patients: they have actually developed such techniques as "laughter meditation," which is described in the September 1995 issue of *Patient Education and Counseling* (Vol. 26, Nos. 1–3, pp. 367–71).

This technique involved a structured exercise of fifteen minutes, divided into three stages: stretching, laughing, and silence. The author says that this approach can be used with other types of therapy to increase the ability to cope with various problems. The author reports that participants' responses vary from deep relaxation, to a feeling of being "whole," to a feeling of being "unburdened," to a feeling of acceptance.

Rx Response
The Indian Laughing Club

Bombay, India, the nation's financial center, is known as "stress city." To relieve the tension, a number of "laughing clubs" have formed—inspired by a physician, Madan Kataria, who has popularized an ancient yoga breathing technique that emphasizes laughing.

He began with a small group that began to tell jokes, and soon, the number had swelled to fifty. Before long more than a hundred "laughing clubs" had appeared around India.

The routine follows this pattern: the group lines up in straight rows and does some stretching. Then, they begin to laugh. The initial snickers are executed so as to encourage deep breathing. Then, they finish up the exercise by jumping about, slapping palms, and laughing so hard that they begin to perspire.

Advanced practitioners can reportedly perform special laughs: the silent "joker laugh," the closed-lips "etiquette laugh," or the huge "Bombay laugh."

What are the benefits?

Participants claim that they are able to shed inhibitions, build self-confidence, breathe more easily—and even give up smoking.

Dr. Kataria also reports that the practice can lower high blood pressure, relieve arthritis, and help with migraine headaches. (See *The Wall Street Journal,* Sept. 12, 1996, p. B1.)

HIDDEN ENERGY SOURCE 4: ADVANCED SPIRITUAL DISCIPLINES

Much has been written about how developing a deep spiritual life can help produce emotional and physical healing. I've gone into some detail about the most recent scientific studies on this subject in previous books, and I won't retread that territory here.

But I do want to emphasize a significant benefit of advanced spirituality that is particularly pertinent to the subject of this book—the recovery of the power of youth. I'm referring to the infusion of new energy and personal power into the person who deepens his inner life by pursuing traditional spiritual disciplines.

In general, scientists studying the phenomenon of faith-related healing make a distinction between religion and spirituality. Sometimes, the outward, often superficial observance of religious practices and traditions is associated with "extrinsic" religion, which lacks the power to transform one's inner life, or to effect healing. In contrast, a deep spirituality that produces inner changes is referred to as "intrinsic" spirituality or religious practice.

Also, there is a movement to avoid confusing true spirituality with psychology or traditional medicine. In other words, the faith that transforms one's life must be viewed and evaluated as a separate force or factor. (See *Journal of Family Practice,* Aug. 1992; 35[2]: p. 201; *Nursing Diagnosis,* July 1996; 7[3]: pp. 100–7; *Journal of Advanced Nursing,* Dec. 1997; 26[6]: pp. 1183–8.)

On the other hand, there is also pressure from a number of experts and researchers not to treat the spiritual dimension of life as just another subject that can be analyzed with current scientific methods and tools. In a debate in the *Journal of Advance Nursing,* for instance, one writer took issue with a proposal that placed spirituality into a quasi-medical category of "integrative energy." She argued that spirituality should not be stripped of its meaning in the name of a "spurious scientism." She recommended that spirituality not be reduced to "acceptable scientific terms," but rather, that nurses be given the chance to study spiritual matters in their historical, literary, and philosophical context. (See issues of Feb. 1997; 25[2]: pp. 282–9; and Oct. 1995; 22[4]: pp. 808–15.)

One of the main markers of the benefits of spirituality, which has emerged in recent studies, is frequent attendance at religious services. For example, a 1997 report in the *American Journal of Public Health* (June 1997; 87[6]: pp. 957–61) revealed that going to church regularly can result in a longer life.

The researchers, who were from the Human Population Laboratory, California Public Health Foundation, Berkeley, followed more than fifty-two hundred residents of Alameda County, California, for twenty-eight years. The frequent attendees, especially the females, had lower mortality rates than the infrequent attendees. Also, frequent service attendees were more likely to stop smoking, increase exercising, increase social contacts, and stay married.

The researchers concluded that the lower mortality rates for those who went to services often could be explained in part by their improved health practices, increased social contacts, and more stable marriages.

In another important pair of studies at Duke and Yale universities, both of which were funded by the National Institute on Aging, scientists found a variety of health benefits. In the Yale project, for instance, more than twenty-eight hundred elderly subjects were followed over a twelve-year period. The researchers found that the participants who attended religious services regularly were more likely to have better physical functional ability later in life (or in our terms, a greater dose of the "power of youth"!). They also discovered that the religious people had stronger social support systems, more optimism, and fewer symptoms of depression. (See *Journal of Gerontology B, Psychological Sciences and Social Sciences,* Nov. 1997; 56[6]: pp. S294–305, and S306–16.)

In the Duke study, those who regularly attended religious services displayed stronger immune systems than those who didn't attend. In fact, the attendees were twice as likely to have strong immune systems. (See *International Journal of Psychiatry Medicine,* 1997; 27[3]: pp. 233–50.)

The import of these and related studies seems clear: regular pursuit of religious disciplines, such as service attendance and prayer, will increase the likelihood that you'll remain vigorous and healthy, well into old age.

To help you develop a personal program that will deepen your spirituality, let me suggest a few practical steps. First, evaluating yourself in the "Spiritual Health" column on the Cooper Energy Scale, which is described in Chapter 3, will give you a good, basic idea about where you stand in your own spirituality.

But more is required. These days, health professionals, who have been impressed with the impact of spirituality on health, are developing increasingly sophisticated guidelines for assessing spiritual needs. Among other things, they have developed means for taking a person's "spiritual history," much as an ordinary physician or nurse would take a personal and family medical history. Typically, they begin with several major areas of concern, including:

- the person's concept of God
- sources of strength and hope
- significance of religious practices and rituals in the individual's life
- perceived relationship between spiritual beliefs and the state of health, including spiritual beliefs as coping mechanisms
- relationship between faith and personal relationships

Then, they develop a series of detailed questions that help them evaluate the strength of the patient's inner life. The way a person answers the questions will help them predict the impact of that person's spirituality on preventing disease, healing, or coping with the pain and discomfort of chronic illness. (See *Archives of Family Medicine*, Jan. 1996; 5[1]: pp. 11–6; *Nursing Clinics of North America,* Sept. 1987; 22[3]: pp. 603–11.)

Because the spiritual dimension is so important to health—yet so hard to quantify—I'd suggest that, in addition to evaluating yourself on the Energy Scale, you take two further steps. First, you should put together your own spiritual history, and second, you should keep tabs on a daily basis on how you are doing spiritually, using what I call a Spiritual Monitor.

Take Your Personal Spiritual History

On a separate pad or computer document, perhaps where you have begun to record your Energy Scale, begin to write up your personal spiritual history. Here's a suggested outline that you might follow:

- Identify the point or period when faith or the spiritual dimension of life became important to you. Be as precise and detailed as possible, including dates, your feelings, and others who may have been involved. Also, describe specific changes that may have occurred in your inner life, your moral views, and your social interactions.

- State the major milestones in your spiritual journey. Include special insights, spiritual breakthroughs, and renewal experiences. Again, be specific, and describe your feelings and changes that occurred in your inner life and outward practices.

- Describe situations in which your faith has made a significant difference in your health and energy levels.

- What do you believe are the outer limits of faith-based healing or health enhancements—even if you haven't yet experienced or witnessed these phenomena? Don't hold back here. If you believe miracles are possible, say so. Studies have demonstrated that the healing power of even the placebo effect—which is not supernatural—is rooted in the ability to believe. Furthermore, increasing numbers of physicians recognize the power of faith.

- Give details of the spiritual disciplines or practices you currently observe. Examples include attendance at religious services, personal prayer, Bible or theological studies, healing sessions, volunteer work, service to the needy, and small "share" group meetings.

With this spiritual history in hand, you now have a better picture of the inner journey you've taken over the years. You can see where you've made progress, and what areas of your spiritual life still need work.

Using the Spiritual Monitor

Now, you're ready to take the second step in determining your current spiritual condition—evaluating yourself at least once a week with the accompanying "Spiritual Monitor."

This self-evaluation, which is reminiscent of the spiritual assessments done at a growing number of hospitals and clinics, has been designed to dovetail with the Cooper Energy Scale in Chapter 3. In fact, I would suggest that you use this Spiritual Monitor every time you do a self-evaluation with the Energy Scale. Your answers on the Monitor can be transferred, in summary form, directly to the right-hand column, "Spiritual Health," on the Energy Scale.

SPIRITUAL MONITOR

Spiritual Discipline	Peak	High	Average	Low	Zero
Private Prayer/ Meditation					
Bible/ Spiritual Study					
Support Group/ Prayer- Share					
Family Relations					
Service to Needy					
Charitable Giving					
Worship/ Religious Services					
Giving Spiritual Guidance to Others					

Those readers who have devoted years to nurturing their spiritual lives will immediately recognize this Spiritual Monitor as a "bare-bones" attempt to outline the disciplines and concerns of the spiritual life. Also, I readily admit that as a practicing Christian myself, I'm sure I haven't been able to avoid some built-in biases toward my own faith and its requirements for spiritual growth. On the other hand, this Monitor should at least prove helpful as a starting point, to get you thinking about the state of your inner life, and what you may need to do to strengthen it.

Now, let me say a word about quantity as opposed to quality in evaluating your spiritual life. Clearly, going to religious services every week, or even praying every day, won't automatically make you a deeply spiritual person. Still, some of the medical studies I've cited—and a number I haven't mentioned—emphasize the importance to physical health and emotional well-being of frequency and regularity in attending religious services and other disciplines.

So quantity does count as well as quality—most likely because doing something frequently tends to build good habits, change attitudes, and condition us more effectively. Certainly this principle applies with exercise: we know from multiple studies that regular aerobic workouts and strength training are what produce the best benefits. Not only that, infrequent physical exercise, say just on the weekends, can actually be dangerous. It would seem wise to apply this understanding analogously to our spiritual fitness.

Finally, here are some guidelines for evaluating yourself with the Monitor:

Private Prayer/Meditation. This spiritual discipline dovetails with the second "hidden" source of energy, finding a "peaceful place." In other words, when you've found some solitude, it's important to fill it with relaxing content. I mentioned gardening as one possibility under the peaceful-place discussion. But many will find private prayer or meditation to be even more helpful as a means of reducing stress, enhancing their spiritual lives, and infusing themselves with more youthful energy.

I won't attempt to suggest specific types of private prayer; there are many devotional guides that can do a better job than I can. But I will reiterate my point about the importance of devoting a minimum quantity of time to this practice. In my own life, I've found that it takes about a half hour per day to begin to reap significant benefits from prayer and meditation, and many spiritual counselors would recommend an hour or more per day.

Bible/Spiritual Study. Faith must have content, and for this reason, I strongly recommend that you get into a regular theological or Bible study at your place of worship. Seeing how the spiritual life has been nurtured since ancient times—and also learning from history about the moral and spiritual mistakes of others—is an essential part of spiritual maturity.

Support Group/Prayer-Share. A fully developed religious experience can never be an insular, solitary affair. To be sure, regular one-on-one encounters with God are essential. But plugging into a like-minded community is also essential for advice, correction, and training in spiritual growth.

Often, the most effective support groups and "prayer-and-share" cells that have arisen from broader faith communities consist of about four to eight people who meet, share, and pray together regularly. The small size encourages more individual participation, freedom, and opportunity for personal growth. One of the most famous models for this type of group would be the New Testament "share and support group" consisting of Jesus, Peter, James, and John.

Family Relations. Here, you should evaluate how well you're getting along with each of your family members. These relationships always involve a moral dimension, just as the family itself is widely regarded as a fundamental cultural institution with deep spiritual roots.

Service to Needy. Spiritual growth traditionally implies a growing sense of duty to those who are less fortunate. I know that in my busy professional and family life, it's easy to overlook my obligation to reach beyond my personal circle to help others. One factor that helps me is my medical training: many times someone in dire physical or emotional need will cry out to me for help. In anticipation of such cases, I've always tried to follow a "good Samaritan" policy to respond immediately when I perceive such a need. But to stay sensitized in this area, it's advisable to check your score on this particular line at least once a week.

Charitable Giving. There is a strong tradition in both Christian and Jewish theology of giving out of one's financial means to those in need. The tithe, or one-tenth of income, is emphasized heavily in the Old Testament, and sacrificial giving is highlighted many times in the New Testament.

I make a distinction here between giving of your material goods and giving of yourself. The previous line, "Service to Needy," involves a sacrifice of time and emotional energy. In many ways, this time commitment is more demanding than the financial commitment—but both are essential for a well-rounded spiritual life.

Worship/Religious Services. I've already cited a variety of scientific studies that show how going regularly to religious services can translate into better health, a stronger immune system, and greater stores of youthful vigor and staying power, well into old age. Many times we associate regular worship attendance with old-fashioned, outdated practices that are destined to go the way of the country church or the hellfire preachers. But in fact, evidence is accumulating to show that the old ways are the best ways—at least in terms of being able to produce total health and well-being.

For example, a 1998 review in the *Archives of Family Medicine* (Vol. 7, pp. 118–24) found that 80 percent of the scientific reports assessed indicated a positive link between religion and good health. One five-year study showed that men who attended church once a week had a 40 percent lower risk of death from heart disease than those who worshiped less often.

Giving Spiritual Guidance to Others. The great Greek tragedian Sophocles wrote in his *Trachiniae*, "One must learn by doing the thing; for though you think you know it, you have no certainty, until you try" (translated by Sir George Young).

I'd go one step further by saying, "One must learn by teaching the thing."

In the spiritual realm, personal maturity and progress often come most quickly when we convey what we know to others, and perhaps help them begin to follow the path we have chosen. Also, as we communicate our insights, others may begin to enjoy the benefits of the vigor and emotional health that often accompany a deep spirituality. For evidence, see the accompanying box, which shows how deeply religious mothers, who pass on their faith, can reduce their children's risk of depression.

Rx Response
Can a Mother's Religion Protect Her Children from Depression?

The answer to this question is apparently "yes," according to a 1997 report in the *Journal of the American Academy of Child and Adolescent Psychiatry* (Oct. 1997; 36[10], pp. 1416–25).

Researchers from the Department of Psychiatry, College of Physicians and Surgeons, Columbia University, followed 60 mothers and 151 of their offspring over a ten-year period. During that time, they assessed the "religiosity" of both the mothers and the children on the basis of several factors: the importance of religion in their lives, the frequency of their attendance at religious services, and their affiliation with a religious denomination.

The investigators found two main factors, the religiousness of the mothers and the concordance, or agreement, of religious commitments between mother and child, which protected the children from depression. Also, this protective influence operated independently of other factors, such as maternal bonding, the social function of the mother, or maternal demographics (where the mother lived).

Finally, here's a practical word about how to do a spiritual self-assessment according to the five levels of spiritual well-being, from "peak" to "zero," indicated on the vertical columns of the Monitor:

If you find you score in the "peak" or "high" category for any discipline, you're probably doing all right in that area. On the other hand, if you're only "average"—and certainly if your self-assessment is "low" or "zero"—you should pay some attention to strengthening your weaknesses.

This discussion of the four "hidden" or "secret" sources of personal energy concludes our basic introduction to the power of youth—and to the targeting strategies that can promote that vigor, energy, and can-do attitude that you may have feared you had lost forever.

In the second part of this book, we'll take a closer look at how various targeting strategies can be used effectively to overcome specific challenges of the major age-groups that may be represented in your household.

But before we move on to Part 2, one other important issue remains—an issue that in many ways can determine just how effectively you'll be able to develop specific targeting strategies. I'm referring to your ability to evaluate and make practical use of new medical findings that seem to make the news every day. To figure out the true meaning of these reports, it's frequently necessary to cut through considerable medical confusion, so that you can get to the heart of those medical studies that are really useful, and identify those you would do well to ignore.

6

· · · · · · · · · · · · ·

Cutting Through the Medical Confusion

Some of the most common complaints I hear from audiences when I deliver one of my talks on health and well-being go like this:

"Dr. Cooper, how can I know what to believe about medical advice and guidelines? There are just too many contradictory reports."

"One day, I hear fat in my diet is bad; the next day, I hear it's good."

"I hear from one expert that large doses of antioxidant vitamins are helpful, but then the next expert tells me they're harmful."

"Somebody says that vigorous exercise is essential. But somebody else says that light exercise is all I need—or that exercise is not important at all."

"It's all so confusing. Sometimes, I just think maybe I should forget all the medical advice and reports I'm hearing and do whatever I feel like doing."

I can sympathize because—despite my roles as practicing physician, chairman of a major international research institute, and spokesman for the international preventive medicine movement—I wrestle with much of the same confusion that you do. The main difference between us is that because of my position, I am confronted with an overriding responsibility to cut through the confusion—and find those fundamental principles of good health that are likely to stand up in the future under the toughest scientific scrutiny.

In this chapter, I want to pass on some insights and analytical tools that will help you escape the quagmire of conflicting reports that have a bearing on your health, yet may have been immobilizing you. Our goal will be threefold:

- to develop tools that will enable you to pinpoint and cut through the medical confusion in your life
- to find those promising reports that are probably worth following
- to identify the bedrock principles that must be observed

Now, let's take a look at the first objective—to pinpoint the medical confusion that you are confronting, and find ways of cutting through it.

MAKING SENSE OF THE MEDICAL MAZE

I must confess that sometimes I do get frustrated when a particular health report seems to contradict another recent report on the same subject. But my final response is not to throw up my hands and walk away from the issue. Instead, I begin to evaluate the confusing or contradictory information by applying some rather simple, but quite powerful analytical tools.

Here are some of the key questions I ask to help me put each of the conflicting studies or reports into proper perspective. See if these queries can help you cut through the confusion as well.

Was the study done on humans or animals? Human studies always carry more weight than animal studies if you're trying to determine whether a set of scientific findings may apply to you.

Putting rodents on a near-starvation diet, for instance, may help them to live longer, as some research has demonstrated. But that doesn't necessarily mean that the same sort of diet is appropriate for you. Animal studies always have to be tested in some way on a human population to see whether the findings are transferable.

How many people participated in each study? If there were thousands of subjects—as in the studies that have been done by Dr. Ralph Paffenbarger on the health condition of nearly seventeen thousand Harvard alumni—the report will carry more weight than if there were only a handful.

How many years did the research study? "Longitudinal" studies—that is, those that involve following subjects over many years—are usually more valuable than studies done on a one-shot basis or over a relatively short period of time, such as five years or less.

There are several reasons for this fact. First, if a drug or nutritional supplement is being tested, health benefits may not become evident until several years have elapsed. Second, long-term side effects may not show up immediately.

Third, if scientists are investigating risk factors for various slow-building diseases, such as heart disease and cancer, decades may be required to reach definitive conclusions. One of the most famous examples of such research is the Framingham project, conducted by scientists from Harvard and other leading medical institutions in Framingham, Massachusetts.

Finally, the ultimate impact of certain lifestyle habits—such as exercise or taking special nutritional supplements, like vitamins—may take decades. In studies involving the database we have amassed at the Cooper Institute for Aerobics Research, for instance, scientists have been able to determine that moderate exercise has a dramatically beneficial influence on death rates from all causes. Obviously, however, to conduct such a study, you have to follow the subjects long enough so that some begin to complete their full life span.

Who were the participants—and what was the condition of their health? If you are trying to determine the applicability of a study to you or your loved ones, it's important to ascertain as precisely as possible the personal characteristics of the study participants.

For example, you should find out such facts as these:

- age range of the subjects
- their gender
- state of their health (Are they completely healthy without medical symptoms, or are they cardiac patients, diabetics, or in some other category?)
- their physical condition (Are they sedentary, moderately fit, or elite athletes?)
- their lifestyle habits (Are they nonsmokers, smokers, light drinkers, or heavy drinkers?)

The reason this information is so important is fairly obvious: the closer the subjects are to you in their personal characteristics, the more likely it is that the findings in the study will apply to you.

So suppose that some researchers have conducted a study of obese, sedentary, middle-aged men, who have very low HDL ("good") cholesterol, a family history of early heart attacks, and a personal history of angina pains. Predictably, the investigators have concluded that these subjects are at high risk for heart attacks.

If you are a fifty-year-old man with many of these characteristics, then you should take notice, because you are at risk. But if you are a thirty-year-old athletic woman with high levels of HDL cholesterol and no family history of heart trouble, you are very unlikely to face a problem with your heart anytime soon. So the study probably won't have any immediate or direct application to you.

Did a recognized, reputable organization or research group conduct the study? Far too many people I encounter these days—including many members of the medical profession—begin to take supplements or herbs, or submit to unorthodox procedures simply because they have heard something positive about the unsubstantiated approach from an acquaintance, or read about a healing in some popular magazine.

For example, one quite intelligent, highly educated executive reported that he had been taking the herb lobelia, which he had heard about from a colleague. What he liked about the substance was that it operated as a stimulant to "pick him up" when he was tired, and sometimes, he even experienced a mild "high" feeling. In addition, the man claimed that he had been able to think much more clearly and on the whole, seemed happier about life.

Unfortunately, he was unaware of the downside of lobelia: excessive doses can lower blood pressure, increase heart rate—and may even produce coma and death. But as with most herbs, it was impossible to determine the precise potency of the doses he was taking because of a lack of government regulation of these products.

His physician pointed out these dangers to him—and also suggested that he check the evaluation of this herb in my *Advanced Nutritional Therapies* (Thomas Nelson Publishers, 1996). But the executive departed leaving the impression that he planned to rely on anecdotes from friends and personal experimentation, rather than on solid medical facts.

I'm far too cautious for this sort of approach to herbs, supplements, or any quasi-medical procedures—mainly because I regard my own body and the bodies of my patients, friends, and loved ones as too valuable for experimentation. I may recommend a new approach to treatment if there is at least one solid, broad-based study from a major medical school or a well-recognized research institute. But in most cases, I'll want to see several human studies—and be quite clear in my mind about the risks of side effects—before I'll jump on any novel medical bandwagon.

An example of my relatively cautious approach is the position I've taken in my *Antioxidant Revolution* and *Advanced Nutritional Therapies,* which suggest that most people should take relatively high doses of certain vitamins. It's true that some have criticized me for making these recommendations before more definitive scientific studies were available. But in fact, I made sure before publishing any of my conclusions that I had the support of dozens of solid studies of humans by leading medical schools and other research institutions.

Was the study published in a reputable, peer-reviewed medical or scientific journal? As a general rule, the only medical findings that you should allow to influence your health habits are those that have been reported in topflight medical or scientific journals. This means publications like the *New England Journal of Medicine*, the *Journal of the American Medical Association, Circulation, Lancet*, or the like. If the article or report you are reading or hearing about fails to mention any such authority, disregard it—or at least wait to act until you have more solidly grounded medical information.

How does the study compare to conflicting studies, and what are the opinions of detached experts who were not involved in the study? If the weight of authority seems clearly to support the current study, then by all means, adjust your personal health habits accordingly. But if the authorities or arguments on both sides of the issue seem about even, assume a wait-and-see strategy.

If there are five studies that support taking a particular supplement—but five more that recommend against it—I would almost always assume a wait-and-see stance.

On the other hand, if you encounter a dozen studies that support one side of a medical position, and only one study that opposes that position, the reasonable approach is to go with the majority position.

Another related test that you can use is to check the response among those medical or scientific experts who were not involved in the research. If most outside authorities question the results of the study, that's a good reason not to use it as a basis for changing your health practices—at least not until the findings have been confirmed or replicated by another group of researchers. On the other hand, if most of the scientific community seems quite impressed with the new study, it may very well be worth following, despite the fact that it runs counter to previous medical knowledge.

Here's an illustration of how this process may work:

A wide variety of studies have shown health benefits for taking at least 400 IU per day of natural vitamin E supplements. The likely benefits include the reduction in the risk for various cancers, cataracts, and heart disease. One study, however, suggested that taking relatively large doses of vitamin E through supplements may suppress the body's natural ability to produce antioxidants.

Would this particular study be sufficient to warrant my recommending that the taking of vitamin E supplements be halted?

Certainly not—mainly because the overwhelming weight of scientific evidence supports the continued use of vitamin E supplements. Of course, I would certainly recommend that we keep an eye out for studies that may be able to duplicate or expand upon the conflicting study. But my expectation is that this study will prove to have limited, if any, bearing on my recommendations, and those of many other researchers, for taking 400 IU—or in some instances, even higher daily doses—of vitamin E.

Do the details of the study support the conclusion suggested in the headlines? A major mistake many people make is to listen to a brief TV announcement about a new study that's just been released—or perhaps glance quickly at a news headline or news "lead" (the first sentence or two)—and then draw a hasty conclusion. Most misconceptions and confusion arise from failing to dig deeply enough into the story.

A recent report by the Associated Press, which was published by America Online on the Internet, carried a headline that made one of my patients do a double take: "Smoking May Lower Some Cancer Risks."

If a cigarette smoker reads only this headline, his first reaction may be to light up—and to forget any thoughts about quitting a cigarette habit. After all, one of the main reasons you're supposed to stop smoking is to reduce your risk of cancer. Yet now we seem to be hearing that the opposite is true—that you may actually reduce the risk by continuing to smoke!

My advice: keep on reading!

If you did move carefully through this particular story, you would have discovered what the writer actually said:

A small group of women—those with particular gene mutations linked to high rates of breast cancer—were able to lower their risk of that disease by smoking cigarettes. Apparently, something in the smoke protected them. Moreover, the researchers discovered that the more they smoked, the lower their risk became.

But the researchers, who published their findings in the May 20, 1998, issue of the *Journal of the National Cancer Institute,* emphasized several caveats in their report.

First, they warned that smoking would significantly increase the risk of other, more dangerous cancers, such as those of the lung, throat, and pancreas. (Also, as we know from other studies, smoking greatly increases the risk of heart disease, emphysema, and other health problems.)

Second, the researchers who conducted the study stated that they wanted other scientists to test their data, just to confirm that what they had found was correct.

Third, they called for more research that might produce a drug that would protect against this special form of breast cancer—but without the serious health risks of smoking.

What this particular illustration boils down to is this: first of all, be sure you read the entire article, or other articles covering the same subject. Don't just stop at the headline or lead. Also, evaluate the standing of the medical authority behind the story. In this instance, there was good reason for confidence because the source was a respected publication of the National Cancer Institute.

Next, if you find that the first newspaper, radio, or TV report seems incomplete, by all means go to another source. For example, you can often find excellent, in-depth reports on new medical findings in comprehensively reported national newspapers like *The New York Times*.

If you still aren't satisfied, check the original medical journal article out of the library, or see if you can find an abstract of the findings on the Internet. The free Web site of the U.S. National Library of Medicine is one option that may be useful.

By posing these questions when you encounter medical confusion, you should be able to make more intelligent decisions about whether you can, or cannot, rely on specific news reports to influence your health habits. Now, let me get you started in this process by suggesting some specific guidelines on several key medical issues.

First, we'll focus on what I've called "promising practices," which are definitely worth following, but which will most likely have to be modified and adjusted as additional scientific evidence becomes available. Then, we'll look at the "bedrock principles," which you must observe if you hope to enjoy a long and healthy life.

Some Promising Practices Worth Following

A number of widely followed health practices are backed up by solid scientific evidence—but are still the subject of considerable inquiry. Even though the final word isn't yet in on these issues, in my opinion we are close enough to certainty for you to make these a part of your health arsenal.

Take Relatively High Daily Doses of Antioxidants

Research is still proceeding on the impact of taking relatively high doses of such vitamins as C, E, and beta-carotene, and minerals such as selenium. But I'm convinced that we know enough right now to support the recommendations I've included in my *Advanced Nutritional Therapies* and *Antioxidant Revolution.*

Specifically, this means that the average adult should be taking daily doses of at least 1,000 mg of vitamin C, 400 IU of vitamin E, 25,000 IU of beta-carotene, and 100 mcg (micrograms) of selenium. (For more precise doses according to age, gender, and exercise level, see the recommendations in the previously mentioned books.)

But even as I make these recommendations, ongoing studies are making it necessary to reevaluate my position. For example, some studies of beta-carotene have indicated that it's best to take in this precursor to vitamin A through the diet, rather than through supplements. The studies suggest that this advice is particularly applicable to heavy smokers and heavy drinkers.

So for beta-carotene, I agree that it's preferable to eat a sweet potato, a medium-size carrot, or a half cantaloupe instead of taking a tablet. But if you can't get enough beta-carotene through your diet, you should definitely include supplements in your regimen—unless you are a smoker, you are an alcoholic, or you have imbibed an alcoholic drink within a few hours before or after you take the supplement.

Note: I highly recommend that you try to take in as much of your daily antioxidant requirements as possible through your foods, rather than through supplements. Unfortunately, some antioxidants, including the all-important vitamin E, can't be obtained in the levels that you need them through foods alone. So supplements must remain an option.

In contrast to the beta-carotene findings, I haven't been quite as impressed by another study, a report on vitamin C in the British journal *Nature* in April 1998. Under such newspaper headlines as "Vitamin C in High Doses May Hurt," and "Study Finds Peril in Taking High Vitamin C Supplement," this report called into question the ingestion of 500 mg or more of vitamin C per day. British researchers at the University of Leicester, who conducted the investigation, reported that 500 mg of the vitamin could produce both benefit and harm to the DNA (genetic programming) of human genes.

But let's look before we leap here. As I've suggested with any such report, let's subject this study to some of the questions you should ask of every new medical study.

First, how many people participated in the study—and over how long a period were they evaluated?

The study was done on only thirty men and women over a six-week period. That's not exactly an overwhelming sample to justify overturning all the good things we know about vitamin C supplementation.

Second, who were the participants, and what was the state of their health and fitness?

The reports I've read on the British team's findings make no reference to the precise nutritional or fitness status of the participants. They were identified as "healthy," but several unanswered questions come to my mind.

For example, how much vitamin C were the subjects taking in through their diets? Is it possible that the cells of any of the participants were already saturated with vitamin C because of a high intake of such foods as orange juice? If so, the supplements would have been much more likely to operate negatively, as pro-oxidants.

Also, how much exercise, if any, were the participants doing each week? My own recommendations on vitamin C intake distinguish between those who are physically very active, and those who are only moderately active or sedentary. The reason for this distinction is that vitamin C and other nutrients have a tendency to wash out of your body as you perspire. The more you sweat, the more antioxidants you are likely to lose—and the more you need to take in, either through your diet or through supplementation. Also, smokers need more vitamin C.

Third, what do other experts say about the study?

One of the news reports I read did an excellent job of exploring the other side of this story. In this account, several experts in the antioxidant field responded that the mixed results of the British study show that it should not be regarded as definitive on the vitamin C issue. They said that more research is required before any final conclusions can be drawn—and I certainly agree.

Are there any pluses for the study—and should it be given any weight in our personal fitness and nutritional programs?

The British researchers do seem to have expanded our understanding about the so-called "pro-oxidant" qualities of antioxidants.

Note: The term *pro-oxidant* as used here refers to the fact that in some cases, an antioxidant like vitamin C or vitamin E when taken in large doses may begin to work in a way opposite to how it's supposed to behave.

Antioxidants in the bloodstream are supposed to protect cells and their DNA from damage from free radicals, which are unstable oxygen molecules in our bodies that have been associated with cancers, atherosclerosis, and other diseases. But sometimes, when there is too much of a particular antioxidant, it may become neutral in its operations, or may even begin to damage DNA. This destructive action, which the British workers said they identified in the small sample of people they studied, is something we need to monitor as we set limits on antioxidant intake in the future.

One constructive way to do this, according to the British researchers, is to obtain our vitamin C from foods, such as orange juice, cranberry juice cocktail, or cantaloupe, rather than through supplements. The reason, they say, is that foods containing vitamin C have shown no tendency to operate as pro-oxidants.

Certainly, I've agreed with this basic position in all my writing on the subject of antioxidants. Whenever possible, we should take in our daily dose of antioxidants through food. It's quite possible to obtain 1,000 milligrams of vitamin C per day through the diet. In fact, if you do rely wholly or primarily on your diet for this vitamin, you'll get much more nutritional value than you will from any supplement.

So if you are a person who is involved in moderate or light physical exercise—and you can ingest that much through orange juice, cantaloupe, broccoli, and other such foods—then by all means do so. But for most of us, and especially heavy exercisers, who need 1,500–2,000 mg of vitamin C per day, some supplementation will be necessary.

At this point, then, the weight of scientific evidence suggests that the potential benefits of vitamin C supplements for fighting free radicals and decreasing the risks of cancers and other diseases far outweigh the possible negative effects suggested by this one limited study.

Using Alternative Medicine Therapies

According to a 1998 survey conducted by InterActive Solutions of Grand Rapids, Michigan, for Landmark Health Care, Inc., 42 percent of American households say they now make use of some type of alternative health care. Illustrations include herbal therapy (17 percent of Americans), chiropractic therapy (16 percent), massage therapy (14 percent), vitamin therapy (13 percent), and a variety of other techniques—including homeopathy, yoga, acupressure, acupuncture, biofeedback, hypnotherapy, and naturopathy. (See *The New York Times*, April 28, 1998, p. B10.)

There has also been growing support among health professionals for the use of alternative medicine techniques, such as prayer and meditation to reduce stress and stress-related conditions, like hypertension. For example, the Oxford Health Plans, Inc., a huge HMO (health maintenance organization), offers such alternative treatments as acupuncture. Also, an estimated thirty medical schools offer courses in alternative medicine.

I'm all for including some of these practices as part of a complete preventive medicine package—and I've recommended a number of them in previous books. At the same time, you should evaluate and judge these approaches at least as strictly as you do the techniques of conventional medicine. Some recent challenges to alternative healing techniques have highlighted how important it is not to allow these claims to go unexamined.

For example, a nine-year-old Colorado fourth grader, Emily Rosa, conducted a highly publicized study on therapeutic touch for her fourth-grade science fair. Therapeutic touch, by the way, doesn't involve actual physical touch. Rather, it relies on the hand-manipulation by healers of supposed "energy fields," which are said to emanate from the bodies of patients. As the healer "adjusts" the fields, medical problems are reportedly relieved or cured.

Emily's study, which was published in the April 1, 1998, issue of the prestigious *Journal of the American Medical Association (JAMA)*, focused on whether twenty-one practitioners of the technique could detect the presence of one of her hands without actually seeing it. As they put their hands through holes that had been cut in a screen, Emily would move her own hand to within a few inches of the right or left hand of the healer.

Significant numbers of the practitioners failed the test. In fact, overall they were able to identify the correct location of Emily's hand no more than 44 percent of the time. (If they had guessed, they would have been right about half the time.)

Predictably, therapeutic healers around the country, numbering in the tens of thousands, were outraged at the study. Among other objections, they argued that the American Medical Association, which publishes *JAMA,* is biased and has an ax to grind with alternative medicine therapies. Also, some said that the technique involves more than just sensing an energy field; emotional and "intuitive" evaluations of the patient are also required.

However this controversy eventually comes out, it points to an ongoing set of issues for alternative therapies. To be sure, some of the techniques do work and should be included as part of a complete healing or preventive medicine program. But each specific approach must be tested and evaluated by scientific studies and analysis. If a particular therapy can't stand up to the test, then members of the medical establishment—as well as the general public—are entirely justified in discarding it.

Limit Your Intake of Filtered Coffee

For as long as I can remember, questions have been raised in the medical community about the impact on our health of caffeine intake, and especially coffee drinking, which is the most common way that adults get their caffeine. Yet the results of various studies have been mixed, with the weight of authority seeming to come down on the side of safety—so long as caffeine is ingested in small daily doses.

Here are some of the salient findings:

- The average woman or man should be safe if she or he takes in no more than two cups of moderately strong coffee per day (about 240 mg of caffeine). A personal note: I limit myself to about a half cup of coffee in the morning, just after I arrive at work.
- Taking in more than five to six cups of coffee per day may trigger a higher incidence of heartbeat irregularities, increased blood pressure, shortness of breath, headaches, and other health problems.
- A January 1997 Norwegian study, published in the *American Journal of Clinical Nutrition* (Vol. 65, No. 1, pp. 136–43), found a strong relationship between increased coffee consumption and higher homocysteine levels in the blood. (High homocysteine is an important risk factor for cardiovascular disease, birth defects, and other health problems.) In this study, forty- to forty-two-year-old women who drank nine or more cups of filtered coffee per day had homocysteine levels of 10.5 micromoles per liter, a result that put them in the moderate-risk range for health problems. In contrast, women who didn't drink coffee had an 8.2 reading, which was in the low-risk area.

- Studies have shown that drinking nonfiltered, boiled coffee may raise cholesterol levels.
- Coffee drinking has been linked to loss of the body's calcium through urination—a process that could decrease your bone density and increase the risk of osteoporosis (the disease characterized by thinning of the bone mass).
- Drinking more than about three cups of coffee per day (or 300 mg of caffeine in another form, such as six cups of brewed tea) may reduce a woman's chance to conceive. (According to one 1995 study at Johns Hopkins University, the chances of becoming pregnant may decline by 26 percent.)
- On the positive side, a small to low-moderate intake of caffeine-containing beverages, including filtered coffee, has been shown to increase mental acuity, alertness, and general feelings of well-being.

As you can see, coffee presents us with a mixed bag—some benefits, but also some potentially serious detriments, especially in high dosages. In short, there is some medical confusion about coffee.

But when I apply the tests mentioned earlier for cutting through the confusion, including closely analyzing and weighing the scientific studies, I come to this conclusion: up to two cups of coffee a day are okay for most people, provided the person has no medical reason to avoid it.

Limit or Eliminate Your Intake of Alcohol

In contrast with my approach to coffee, I reach the opposite conclusion with alcohol. Again, there is a degree of medical confusion: alcohol consumption in small to moderate amounts—say a glass or two of wine per day—has been associated with lower rates of heart disease for both men and women.

On the other hand, even moderate drinking—say one drink of any type per day—has been linked to increased risks of breast cancer. Heavy drinking, of course, is associated with many serious health problems, including high blood pressure, stroke, heart disease, certain cancers, and cirrhosis of the liver—not to mention the high incidence of deaths and injuries that occur among those who drink and drive.

So should you drink, or shouldn't you?

With alcohol, I come down on the side of abstinence as my first choice, because the dangers of excessive use can be so much worse than other questionable habits, such as excessive coffee drinking. Also, the benefits of drinking—notably the reduction of heart disease risk, probably through the raising of levels of "good" (HDL) cholesterol—can usually be achieved through other means, such as aerobic exercise.

If you do choose to drink, there is no confusion about the wisest strategy: medical authorities unanimously conclude that you should always be a light drinker. That means fewer than ten drinks per week for men, or six drinks a week for women. (One drink is equal to one 4-ounce glass of wine, one beer, or one cocktail.)

Rx Response
Alcohol, Drugs, and Women Over Sixty

One of the "dark and dirty little secrets" in the medical community has been the epidemic of alcohol and drug abuse among older women. Fortunately, this tragedy has been exposed to the light by a June 4, 1998, report from Columbia University's National Center on Addiction and Substance Abuse.

Researchers on the two-year study found that 7 percent of women age sixty and older—or about 1.8 million individuals—abuse or are addicted to alcohol. Yet less than 1 percent of this group, who need medical treatment, receive it.

Furthermore, 11 percent of these older women, or about 2.8 million people, abuse or are addicted to mood-altering prescription drugs, such as tranquilizers or antidepressants.

The report, entitled "Under the Rug: Substance Abuse and the Mature Woman," noted that alcohol abuse is more likely to be overlooked among older women—for a number of reasons. First of all, they often drink alone. In addition, their children are often reluctant to confront them.

Doctors also often misdiagnose the problem as dementia or depression. The National Center found further that women who consulted a physician were 37 percent more likely than men to be given a prescription for a tranquilizer, and 33 percent more likely to receive an antidepressant.

Other reasons that older women tend not to seek help for their alcohol or drug problems are that they often can't identify with young drug users in institutional detoxification programs, and they are frequently too embarrassed to admit that they have a problem.

(See *The New York Times,* June 5, 1998, p. A10; Associated Press reports, June 4, 1998.)

These, then, are a few examples of principles and findings that may initially present us with some confusion—but which we should usually follow. Others will be mentioned later in this book—such as the emerging strategy of nutrimedicine, which involves the use of foods as "nutriceuticals" to target and treat specific health problems or complaints. Remember: even though you may initially be disconcerted by conflicting findings and reports, in almost every case you'll find a satisfying answer—if you ask the key questions discussed above, which will enable you to cut through the confusion.

On the other hand, medical research has also presented us with some findings that shouldn't cause any confusion at all. A close look at the research should lead any reasonable person to the conclusion that these issues represent bedrock principles that everyone should accept and follow.

SOME BEDROCK PRINCIPLES THAT SHOULD CAUSE NO CONFUSION

Granted, there is a great deal of uncertainty surrounding many new medical findings and recommendations. The conflicting and sometimes contradictory reports can trigger frustration and despair—and make it seem that no principle of preventive medicine is worth following. Here are three common negative responses that I encounter:

- *Confusion:* "One medical finding seems to contradict the other. I feel immobilized."
- *Fear:* "I'm afraid of making the wrong health choice. So maybe I'll just do nothing."
- *Defiance:* "I say, just ignore the medical news! Whenever some doctor or researcher says, 'You must change your life to lower your risks,' the chances are some other expert will come up with a different recommendation next week. So just forget it, and do whatever you want."

The people in this last group—who probably represent the largest single segment that I run into—are caught up in what might be called "medical agnosticism." They assume that we can't know or learn anything useful from the latest scientific research. So the best approach is just to do nothing—and hope for the best.

The fallacy with such attitudes is that they ignore the fact that there are some clear rules—or what I call "bedrock principles" of preventive medicine. These are truths that you really must follow—and that you neglect to your own great peril—because they have been proven beyond any reasonable doubt to have the power to improve your health and increase your longevity.

Here are a few illustrations of some of these bedrock principles:

Bedrock Principle #1: Engage in Regular, Moderate Aerobic Exercise

Over the years, I've become embroiled in a number of disputes over whether exercise is important to health and longevity—and if it is important, how much you should do. At this point, I won't retrace all the studies and arguments that have been set forth in my previous books. But I will say this: *the overwhelming weight of scientific evidence demonstrates conclusively that abandoning a sedentary lifestyle and following a moderate exercise routine will greatly*

*reduce your risk of dying from all causes—and enhance your chance
of living a longer, more active life.*

Here are some of the latest findings that add further support to this
conclusion:

A 1998 report in the *New England Journal of Medicine* concluded
that regular walking over distances of more than two miles per day
was associated with a lower overall death rate among the 707 men,
ages sixty-one to eighty-one, who participated in the study.

The researchers, who were supervising the Honolulu Heart
Program, found that over a twelve-year follow-up period, men who
walked less than one mile per day were nearly twice as likely to die
prematurely as those who walked more than two miles per day.

Overall, the distance walked was inversely related to mortality,
after adjustment was made for various other risk factors. This means
that the farther you walk, the more your risk of dying is reduced. (See
NEJM, Jan. 8, 1998; 338[2], pp. 94–9.)

In a study of twins published in the February 11, 1998, issue of the
Journal of the American Medical Association, researchers from
Helsinki, Finland, found that taking a brisk half-hour walk at least six
times a month was able to cut the risk of death by 44 percent.

The researchers, who evaluated nearly sixteen thousand healthy
male and female twins an average of nineteen years, discovered that
even a twin involved in very light activity (walking fewer than six
times per month) was 30 percent less likely to die than a twin who
was sedentary.

This investigation was particularly important because it afforded
scientists the opportunity to compare two people with similar genes
and heredity. The investigators concluded that the impact of "bad
genes" could be overcome to some extent by regular exercise and
other good health habits.

Doing moderate exercise thirty minutes a day (either in one workout session or collectively in several smaller time increments), preferably almost every day per week, will significantly reduce the risk of
heart disease, high blood pressure, cancer, and diabetes, according to
the U.S. Surgeon General's report released July 12, 1996.

Moderate exercise or activity in this context meant burning at least 150 calories per day through such activities as walking two miles in thirty minutes, bicycling three miles in thirty minutes, or swimming laps for twenty minutes.

This report also allowed for doing the thirty minutes of exercise per day in ten-minute increments—but I must respectfully dissent from this approach. Because the most important studies showing benefits for exercise have measured continuous activity, I recommend that you choose a standard endurance workout that you can do for at least thirty consecutive minutes, such as walking, jogging, bicycling, or swimming.

To put this bedrock principle in practical, programmatic terms, I would make this recommendation: everyone should do at least twenty to thirty minutes of continuous endurance exercise three to four days a week—and preferably more often.

Note: I haven't mentioned strength conditioning in this context, primarily because there are too few studies currently available on the benefits. But as you've already seen, I believe that everyone needs to include a strength and flexibility component in his weekly routine. Furthermore, the evidence is accumulating that the older you are, the more strength and flexibility work you need. (See Chapter 2 and those that follow for my specific views and recommendations on this topic.)

Bedrock Principle #2: Limit Fat Consumption

Your daily intake of fats should amount to no more than 20 to 30 percent of your total calorie consumption. Also, the fats should be consumed in these proportions: at least one-third monounsaturated, one-third polyunsaturated, and no more than one-third saturated.

Without question, the overwhelming weight of scientific authority now tells us to limit our intake of fats and consume the fats we do eat in approximately the proportions suggested above. But as with many other health issues, conflicting reports about fat consumption have caused some public confusion—and that includes a number of my own patients.

A headline in *The Wall Street Journal* (Dec. 24, 1997, p. B8) symbolizes the problem: "The Surprising New Skinny on Fat: It Might Cut Risk of Stroke, Study Finds."

A fat-lover glancing at this headline might be tempted to read no farther. I can hear the comment now: "You see, even the scientists can't make up their minds whether fat is good or bad. So I'll just eat whatever I want."

But remember, to cut through the confusion, you must read farther—and you must read analytically.

If you did continue to read this particular story, you would learn that the report was limited to a rather narrow group: middle-aged men who were free of heart disease at the beginning of the study. Also, experts from the American Heart Association, who were quoted in this article, cautioned that the results need to be confirmed by much larger studies, including both men and women from other age-groups.

In addition, the research for the article was based on what each subject said he had eaten in one twenty-four-hour period. According to my friend Dr. Scott Grundy, chairman of the Department of Human Nutrition at the University of Texas Southwestern Medical School in Dallas, this approach represents a "weak method" of research that should never have been reported to the general public through a newspaper. (See Associated Press report in *The Palm Beach Post,* Dec. 24, 1997, p. 1.)

Finally, and most important, any advantage that fat confers with strokes must be balanced against the well-established evidence that high-fat diets increase the risk of heart disease. And, as the following box shows, the *type* of dietary fat—not just the *amount*—can play a critical role in women.

Heart disease, the AHA experts noted, kills a half million Americans each year, or three times the number of those who die from stroke. So really, this report should cause no confusion at all.

Rather, it just provides us with a little extra information about how fats may interact with a particular disease.

How Does Dietary Fat Influence
Heart Disease Risk in Women?

More than eighty thousand women, ages thirty-four to fifty-nine, were evaluated in the Nurses' Health Study to determine if there was any link between their dietary intake of specific types of fat and their risk of coronary disease, according to a 1997 report in the *New England Journal of Medicine*.

The women in the study had no known coronary disease, history of stroke, cancer, high cholesterol, or diabetes. But after following the women over a fourteen-year period, the researchers identified 939 cases of nonfatal or fatal heart attacks from coronary artery disease.

What might have been the cause of these heart attacks?

The investigators found that each 5 percent increase of energy intake (calories) from saturated fats (such as butter) was associated with a 17 percent increase in the risk of coronary disease. In contrast, the increase in risk of heart disease associated with the intake of monounsaturated fat (such as olive oil) and polyunsaturated fat (such as corn oil) was negligible.

The investigators concluded that replacing saturated fats and "trans unsaturated fats" (those that have been hardened through artificial hydrogenation) with unhydrogenated monounsaturated and polyunsaturated fats would be more effective than reducing overall fat intake in preventing coronary heart disease in women.

The researchers estimated that the replacement of 5 percent of energy intake (calories) from saturated fat with an equivalent amount of unsaturated fats would reduce women's risk of heart disease by 42 percent. Also, they estimated that

> replacing 2 percent of energy intake (calories) from trans
> unsaturated (hydrogenated) fats with unhydrogenated, unsat-
> urated fats would reduce heart disease risk by 53 percent.
> (See *NEJM,* Nov. 20, 1997; 337: pp. 1491–9.)

In the last analysis, medical research proves that our fat consumption—and especially consumption of saturated fats, such as butter—should be limited. Other research by Dr. Grundy and others has
demonstrated that some protection against heart disease is associated
with a "Mediterranean diet," which emphasizes monounsaturated
fats, such as olive oil.

A study published in the January 12, 1998, issue of the *Archives of
Internal Medicine* has given more ammunition to those who advocate
weighing the intake of fats more heavily toward monounsaturated
fats than the other types. The researchers found that women ages
forty to seventy-six who ate monounsaturated fats had a lower risk of
breast cancer than those who ate other types of fat. Also, they suggested that polyunsaturated fats—which are found in such foods as
corn oil, safflower oil, and soybean oil—may actually increase the
risk of breast cancer.

Although these findings are intriguing, Dr. Walter Willett, an epi-
demiologist at the Harvard School of Public Health and a coauthor of
the study, cautioned that the protective effect of the monounsaturated
fat intake might be relatively small. In any event, he said, eating
monounsaturated fats would certainly do no harm—so long as total
fat intake is kept low enough to maintain proper body weight. (See
The New York Times, Jan. 13, 1998, p. B17.)

Clearly, then, even though new information continues to come in on
the impact of fat intake, the above "bedrock principle" remains intact:
limit your fats to no more than 30 percent of your daily calorie consumption. When you do eat fats, whenever possible choose those that
are monounsaturated. By choosing the "mono" type, by the way, you
may get the best of two worlds. That is, you'll be taking in "good" fats
that will not tend to increase your risk of heart disease, and at the same
time you may reduce your risk of stroke and breast cancer.

But what about trans unsaturated fats, or the hardened fats, that can be hidden in your diet? How do you account for and avoid these? The following box tells how to "unmask" these fats.

Energy Pack
Will Hardened Fats Produce Hardened Arteries?

An estimated 5 to 10 percent of the fats in our diet are highly destructive "hidden fats," in the sense that they lurk undetected in many of our foods.

But these substances, which are also known more technically as "trans unsaturated fats," can be unmasked by the alert consumer. One way is to check food labels to see if they say the ingredients include "hydrogenated" or "partially hydrogenated" fats. This type of "trans" fat is produced from polyunsaturated vegetable fats, such as corn oil, by artificial hydrogenation—a process that makes them firmer and more resistant to becoming rancid.

The editors of the prestigious *New England Journal of Medicine* say that you can think of the term *trans* in this kind of fat as being equivalent to the word *hardened.* A good example, they suggest, is the glazed doughnut, though plenty of other "stiff" or "hardened" fatty food products, such as margarine, commercial crackers, and pastries fall into this category.

Can these "hard" fats cause "hardened" arteries, or atherosclerosis?

Cumulative research over the past few years suggests that "trans" or hydrogenated fats may indeed contribute to the risk of coronary heart disease. For example, studies have demonstrated that these fats can raise levels of "bad" (LDL) cholesterol. Also, reports from the Nurses' Health Study have linked "trans" fats to heart disease.

More research is still required for us to reach a definitive

---

decision on the precise, dangerous role of these artificially produced fats. But in my view, enough evidence is available right now for you to watch those food labels and when possible, avoid those with the "hydrogenated" term that signals the presence of trans unsaturated fats. (See *The New England Journal of Medicine,* Nov. 20, 1997; 337: pp. 1544–5.)

Note: To minimize your intake of "trans" fats and still have a spread for your bread or muffin, choose tub margarine or tube-dispensed margarine over stick margarine. Even better, stick to low-fat jellies or other low-fat or nonfat spreads that are not hydrogenated or partially hydrogenated.

Bedrock Principle #3: Avoid Obesity

An important, final, and official word is now in on one of the dangers of obesity: on June 1, 1998, the American Heart Association designated it as a major risk factor for heart attacks, along with smoking, high blood pressure, high cholesterol, and a sedentary lifestyle. Other health conditions that have been associated with obesity include diabetes, hypertension, birth defects, and various types of cancer.

Unfortunately, Americans have a long way to go to overcome this problem. A study published in the May 1998 issue of *Science* found that 54 percent of adults and 25 percent of children are overweight. Other studies have found that as many as 74 percent of Americans twenty-five years old or older are overweight.

What does it mean to be overweight or obese?

Often, obesity is defined as being at least 20 percent above your optimum body weight, or on average carrying an extra twenty-five to thirty-five pounds. Also, a standard we use at the Cooper Clinic is linked to body fat: women under forty carry less than 22 percent body fat in relation to their total weight. Those forty and older should have no more than 26 percent body fat. Men under forty should have less than 19 percent body fat, while those forty and older should carry no more than 20.5 percent body fat.

How to Find the Weight Range That Will Give You Your Ideal Percentage of Body Fat

At the Cooper Clinic, we take precise measurements of our patients' body fat by using a combination of underwater weighing and measurements of fat folds on the body with calipers.

But you can get a general idea of your best weight range, which will give you the right percentage of body fat, just by using this simple formula, which is a modification I've developed on the classic "Mahoney Formula."

For men, your ideal fat percentage range is 15 to 19 percent of your total body weight. Follow these steps to find your weight range in pounds, which will correlate with the proper percentage range:

Step #1: Determine your height in inches.

Step #2: Multiply that number times 4.

Step #3: Subtract 128 from the result in Step #2. This gives you the approximate weight in pounds that represents 15 percent body fat for your size.

Step #4: Multiply the result in Step #3 by 10 percent (0.10).

Step #5: Add the result in Step #4 to the result in Step #3. This gives you the approximate weight in pounds that represents 19 percent body fat for you.

Here's how the formula works in practice for a man. Assume your height is five-foot-nine, or sixty-nine inches. Multiply by four to get 276. Subtract 128 to get 148 pounds—the weight that represents 15 percent body fat for you.

Now, multiply 148 by 0.10 (or 10 percent). That gives you 14.8 pounds. Add that to 148, and you have 162.8 pounds—or the weight that represents 19 percent body fat. This man's ideal weight range, then, would be approximately 148 to 163 pounds.

For women, the ideal range for body fat is 18 to 22 percent. Follow these steps to find your personal weight range:

Step #1: Measure your height in inches.

Step #2: Multiply that result by 3.5.

Step# 3: Subtract 108 from the result in Step #2. That gives you your approximate weight for 18 percent body fat.

Step #4: Multiply the result in Step #3 by 0.10 (10 percent).

Step #5: Add the result in Step #4 to the result in Step #3 to get the weight that represents about 22 percent body fat for you.

Refer to the illustration for men to see how each of these steps can be applied in practice (but remember that the numbers used in each formula are different).

This particular bedrock principle is directly related to the previous one: if you limit your dietary fat intake, you'll automatically limit your calories, and thereby reduce your risk of becoming overweight.

The issue involves some rather simple arithmetic. Carbohydrates (which should constitute about 50 to 70 percent of your daily calorie intake) and protein (which should make up about 10 to 20 percent of your intake) contain many fewer calories than fat. Specifically, 1 gram of carbohydrate or protein translates into about 4 to 5 calories, whereas 1 gram of fat of any type involves about 9 calories.

So if you take in 10 grams of fat in a cookie or some similar food, you'll be adding an extra 90 calories—which will require you to walk or jog about a mile to burn. On the other hand, if you take in 10 grams of carbohydrate in a dish of fat-free yogurt, you'll be adding only forty extra calories.

A word of caution: although it's important to get down to your optimum weight, obesity is only one among a wide array of health concerns. In fact, in a study we did at the Cooper Institute for Aerobics Research in Dallas in 1997, our researchers found that skinny people who were in poor physical condition were more likely to die prematurely than overweight people who exercised regularly.

So the message here is this: get your weight down to the optimum level, but don't forget to follow other bedrock principles of good health!

Bedrock Principle #4: Consume Folic Acid Daily

Although there has been some disagreement about taking vitamin and mineral supplements, there is virtual unanimity in the scientific community about folic acid, which is associated with the B-complex vitamin family. Adults should consume at least 400 micrograms of folic acid daily. The consensus, which was summed up in an April 1998 announcement from a U.S. government-affiliated panel, the Institute of Medicine, may be stated this way:

- All women of childbearing age should take in an extra 400 micrograms of folic acid every day, either as a vitamin supplement or in fortified breakfast cereals or other foods. Reason: protection against birth defects.
- Everyone over age fifty should be taking in at least 400 micrograms of folic acid daily. Reason: protection against coronary disease.

This panel also agreed that amounts of folic acid up to 1,000 mcg per day are acceptable. In addition, they recommended that people over fifty take a supplement of vitamin B_{12} every day—specifically at least 2.4 micrograms per day. They also recommended vitamin B_6, but it should not exceed 100 milligrams per day.

Other studies support my current recommendations on these nutrients: 400 micrograms per day of folic acid for all adults; 50 mg of vitamin B_6; and 400 micrograms of vitamin B_{12}.

In support of my position, here are some of the most recent findings and observations from the medical experts:

- Blood levels of homocysteine—an amino acid that is a strong indicator of heart disease risk—can be lowered significantly by breakfast cereals fortified with folic acid, according to a report in the April 9, 1998, issue of the *New England Journal of Medicine*. The researchers found that cereal providing 499 mcg of folic acid reduced homocysteine blood levels by 11 percent, and cereal with 665 mcg lowered the homocysteine by 14 percent. (See *NEJM* 1998; 338: pp. 1009–15.)

- The author of a 1998 *New England Journal of Medicine* editorial entitled "Eat Right and Take a Multivitamin," stated, "I agree . . . that the evidence that increased consumption of folic acid will prevent cardiovascular disease is strong and that we should recommend consumption of at least 400 mcg of folic acid daily." (April 9, 1998, issue on the Internet, Vol. 338, No. 15, p. 3.)

- Higher intake of folate (generic term for folic acid and related vitamins) is associated with better performance on abstract mental tests, according to a 1997 report in the *American Journal of Clinical Nutrition* (1997; 64: pp. 20–9). Also, according to this study, a higher consumption of vitamins B_6, B_{12}, E, and A has been related to better performance on tests evaluating recall, visual and spatial figures, and abstractions.

Bedrock Principle #5: Eat Fruits and Vegetables

Eat at least five to seven servings of fruits and vegetables—including at least one helping of "cruciferous" vegetables—every day.

This principle dovetails with others, including the intake of antioxidants in the previous section, Bedrock Principle #3 on obesity, and Bedrock Principle #6 on fiber, which follows. In other words, to keep your intake of fiber high and maintain a high intake of antioxidants without gaining weight, you'll have to increase your consumption of vegetables and fruits.

I've highlighted the "cruciferous" vegetables—including broccoli, brussels sprouts, cauliflower, and cabbage (two "B's" and two "C's")—because scientific evidence continues to show that they are particularly powerful in their ability to reduce the risks of cancer, heart disease, diverticulitis, and constipation. (These vegetables are called "cruciferous" because their flowers grow in the form of an X-shaped Greek cross.)

Although most of the important research on these vegetables can be found in my *Advanced Nutritional Therapies,* a more recent report on broccoli is worth mentioning at this point. A study by researchers from Johns Hopkins University, which was published on September 16, 1997, in the *Proceedings of the National Academy of Sciences,* found that broccoli sprouts may be more beneficial than the mature vegetable.

In comparison with mature broccoli, these tender shoots are packed with fifty times more sulforaphane, a powerful anticancer compound. Earlier studies demonstrated that sulforaphane, which is one of the components of broccoli and cauliflower, was instrumental in the production of an enzyme that prevents the development of tumors.

More studies need to be done on broccoli sprouts to confirm these findings. Also, at this writing, the sprouts are not easy to find in commercial food outlets. But if you can find this product, there seems to be nothing to lose, and perhaps a great deal to gain, by adding it to your diet.

Bedrock Principle #6: Include Fiber in Your Diet

Consume at least 20 to 35 grams of fiber per day, with half coming from "insoluble" fiber and half from "soluble" fiber.

If you eat vegetables and fruits in the quantities recommended in the previous Bedrock Principle #5, you should easily reach the 20 to 35 grams-per-day goal of fiber consumption.

Insoluble fiber—which may be found in a wheat bran cereal like All-Bran and vegetables like broccoli—is particularly helpful in protecting against colon cancer, diverticulitis (inflammation of pouches that may develop in the large intestine), and constipation. Soluble fiber—which is contained in oats, apples, citrus fruits, and beans—has also been associated with lowering cholesterol levels.

Because the benefits of insoluble and soluble fiber may vary somewhat, I suggest that you try to orchestrate your diet so that you split your fiber intake equally between the insoluble and soluble types.

Bedrock Principle #7: Stop Bone Loss Through Calcium Intake

Everyone should take in at least 1,000 to 1,500 mg of calcium per day.

Women reach their "peak bone mass" between the ages of about twenty-five and thirty-five. After that, it's all downhill as far as your skeletal system is concerned. The average person loses from about 0.3 to 0.5 percent of bone mass every year after the peak is reached, with the loss accelerating to 2 to 3 percent per year, for a period of eight to ten years, for women who have reached menopause.

The ultimate, catastrophic finale of this steady bone loss is the disease that is the bane of many of the elderly in the United States and other nations as well—osteoporosis. This condition involves the loss of bone density and the increased susceptibility of the bones to fracturing. More than twenty-five million Americans—80 percent of them female—suffer from osteoporosis. Also, this disease results in an estimated 1.5 million hip fractures in the United States each year.

Although it's not possible to stop this steady bone loss completely, the pace at which it occurs can be slowed significantly. Effective preventive strategies include weight-bearing exercise (walking, jogging, calisthenics, and weight training); quitting smoking; upping the dietary intake of calcium; and estrogen intake through hormone replacement therapy (HRT).

In general, all adult women should be consuming 1,500 mg of calcium per day in food plus supplements to make up the difference. Adult men up to age fifty should consume 1,000 mg, and men older than fifty, as well as men of all ages who are heavy exercisers, should be in the 1,000 to 1,200 mg per day range.

Where should you get your calcium?

It's always preferable to get your nutrients through the food in your diet. Good sources include plain yogurt (one cup = 400 mg), skim milk (one 8-ounce glass = 302 mg), and Swiss cheese (one ounce = 272 mg).

Unfortunately, most of us can't get our daily calcium quota through our diets. The average adult takes in only 400 to 600 milligrams of calcium per day, according to a number of studies. Also, even though most adults need three to four servings of calcium-rich foods per day, they get only about two servings. (See *The New York Times,* Aug. 14, 1997, p. 1.)

Why do we do such a bad job of including enough calcium in our diets?

For one thing, many adult diets aren't designed to accommodate enough milk or other dairy products to allow us to make it up to the 1,000 to 1,500 range. We tend to choose coffee, tea, or a soda rather than a glass of skim milk for lunch or a snack.

Also, the older we get, the more likely we are to become "lactose intolerant." This means we have a deficiency of the enzyme lactase, which breaks down milk sugars. Those who lack sufficient supplies of this enzyme may experience considerable discomfort from eating dairy foods, such as excessive gas and diarrhea.

The answer for some of those with lactose intolerance is to experiment with smaller amounts of dairy foods. In other words, there are varying degrees of this condition, and some people may be able to take in limited amounts of milk or yogurt with no ill effects.

It is possible to increase the intake of nondairy calcium-rich foods, such as collards (180 mg per half cup), kale (150 mg per half cup), and broccoli (100 mg per half cup). Unfortunately, however, the calcium imbedded in these vegetables is not as "bioavailable" as that found in dairy products. This means that your body doesn't do as good a job of extracting the calcium from the foods and making use of it.

Another solution for everyone who can't seem to get enough calcium through the diet is to rely on calcium supplements. From the research provided to me by Dr. Charles Pak, director of the Center for Mineral Metabolism and Clinical Research at the University of Texas Southwestern Medical Center in Dallas, I concluded in my *Overcoming Osteoporosis* (Bantam, 1989) that the most effective type is calcium citrate. A number of studies have demonstrated that calcium citrate is more readily absorbed by the body than other calcium supplements.

Bedrock Principle #8: Drink Water

As I said in Chapter 3, not getting enough fluids in your body can be an energy sapper and even a detriment to your health. Because this is a bedrock principle I will repeat the rule again: Drink the equivalent of at least eight 8-ounce glasses of water per day.

Bedrock Principle #9: Don't Smoke

It's been well established that smoking greatly increases the risk of many serious, and often lethal, diseases. These include lung cancer, heart disease, stroke, and osteoporosis. But smoking can lead to other physical disabilities as well, as the following box indicates.

Youth Booster
Can Smoking Cause Hearing Loss?

In a 1998 study funded by the National Institute on Aging, researchers from the University of Wisconsin Medical School evaluated 3,753 adults, ages forty-eight to ninety-two, to determine any link between smoking and hearing loss.

The participants were subjected to standard hearing tests—including otoscopy, screening tympanometry, pure-tone air-conduction, and bone-conduction audiometry. The researchers defined hearing loss as an average loss of more than 25 decibels in the worse ear, as compared with normal hearing. Those who have this level of hearing loss often have trouble understanding conversation when there is background noise.

The researchers found that smokers were 1.69 times as likely to experience hearing loss as nonsmokers. Also, the investigators determined that the more people smoked, the greater their risk of hearing loss. For example, those who smoked an average of a pack a day for forty years were 1.3 times as likely to suffer hearing loss as those who smoked a pack a day for ten years.

Of the total number of participants in the study, 35 percent of the nonsmokers suffered a hearing loss, in contrast to 47

---

percent of ex-smokers and more than 56 percent of current smokers.

The researchers noted that hearing loss affects an estimated 30 to 35 percent of adults, ages sixty-five to seventy-five, in the United States. They also called for further, longitudinal studies (those following a given population over a lengthy period of years) to confirm their findings. (See the *Journal of the American Medical Association,* June 3, 1998; 279: pp. 17–9; and also *USA Today Health,* June 2, 1998; pp. 1–2.)

Unfortunately, according to a study released by the Centers for Disease Control and Prevention in December 1997, nearly 25 percent of American adults continued to smoke in 1995. The researchers observed that the numbers had not changed much since 1990. Among these smokers, 24.5 million were men, and 22.4 million were women, with those who had not graduated from high school constituting a higher proportion than those with more education.

Even as the number of smokers holds steady at a disturbingly high level, the risks for this habit seem to multiply. Here are a few of the most recent findings:

Secondhand smoke poses serious risks to both men and women. According to a May 1998 study published by the American Heart Association's journal *Circulation,* being in a smoke-filled room for only a half hour will trigger the destruction of the blood's antioxidants, which protect us against heart disease by fighting destructive "free radicals."

These free radicals are unstable oxygen molecules that can promote the development of plaque on blood vessels, which is the main cause of atherosclerosis, or "hardening of the arteries." Also, free radicals have been associated with damage to the DNA of cells, a process that may be a precursor to the development of various cancers.

The study by Finnish researchers from Helsinki University Hospital found that nonsmoking men and women who were in the smoke-filled room for a half hour lost about a third of their blood's capacity to neutralize free radicals.

Smoking makes elderly women feel older. In a study published on December 21, 1994, in the *Journal of the American Medical Association,* researchers measured how 9,704 women over age sixty-five performed basic tasks like gripping an object, walking, rising from a chair, and climbing a set of stairs.

They found that in eleven of the twelve categories tested, smokers performed the tasks more poorly than nonsmokers. In fact, according to the researchers, an older woman who smokes may be adding five years to her physiological age. Among other things, elderly women who smoke have significantly lower muscle strength, inferior agility, and worse balance than nonsmokers, according to the report.

In another interesting, but somewhat puzzling issue uncovered by the study, women who were moderate drinkers did better on the physical tasks than their counterparts who were nondrinkers. Specifically, the moderate drinkers—who averaged fewer than fourteen drinks per week—outperformed nondrinkers on eleven of twelve tasks.

But the researchers said that they would not advise an elderly person to start drinking in an effort to improve physical skills. They noted that possible reasons for the superior performance of the drinkers may have included their tendency to be more active socially. Also, they may have been freer than the nondrinkers of physical disabilities. (See *The New York Times,* Dec. 22, 1944, p. A 10; and related Associated Press report.)

Besides making you *feel* older, smoking can also make you *look* older, according to the study in the following box.

Youth Booster
"Does Cigarette Smoking Make You Ugly and Old?"

This question constitutes the title of a 1992 article in the *American Journal of Epidemiology*—and the answer that the authors gave, after perusing five studies over the previous twenty years, was a resounding "yes."

They concluded that the evidence supported the conclusion that smoking causes wrinkling of the skin, which can make smokers appear unattractive and prematurely old. Specifically, cigarette smoke decreases capillary and arteriolar (small artery) blood flow in the skin. This process may damage connective tissues that help maintain the integrity of the skin. (See *American Journal of Epidemiology*, April 15, 1992; 135[8]: pp. 839–42.)

Later confirmation of this conclusion came from a 1995 Spanish study that evaluated the connection among smoking, sun exposure, and aging. After measuring facial wrinkles in 282 healthy subjects, the researchers found a statistically significant, accelerated risk for skin aging in smokers. (See *Rev Clin Esp,* March 1995; 195[3]: pp. 147–9.)

In a study on a related issue, Danish researchers looked into the possible connection between smoking and the degree or deepness of wrinkles on the face. Specifically, they focused on wrinkles just to the outside side of the "canthus," or the outer angle of skin formed by the eyelids.

After studying a random sample of 4,485 women and 2,485 men, ages forty to sixty-nine years, the investigators discovered that for both sexes, the prevalence of deep wrinkles increased with increasing age and with decreasing household income.

But in men, there was an additional factor: They found a significant association between cumulated cigarette consumption and the degree of deep wrinkles. In contrast, the deepness of women's wrinkles wasn't affected by smoking. The researchers speculated that the difference might lie in the men's greater exposure to sunlight, and also the more prevalent use of face creams among the women.

(See *Ugeskr Laeger,* Feb. 25, 1991; 153[9]: pp. 660–2.)

These are just a few of the bedrock principles of preventive medicine that will enable you to regain the power of youth in your life. Obviously, much more needs to be said about recapturing that youthful vigor you once enjoyed—and much more will be said in the ensuing pages. But the main point I want to make at this juncture is this: even though some reports we hear about preventive medicine strategies may seem confusing, there are many important principles that should not confuse us—and that should become basic guidelines for the way we live our lives.

If I could only convince most adult Americans—including many of my own patients!—to follow faithfully both the truly promising medical reports and the bedrock principles of preventive medicine, we would begin to see a revolution in our energy levels and longevity.

The possible shape of such a bright and healthy future has been outlined by Dr. James Fries and a team of Stanford University researchers, who studied 1,741 University of Pennsylvania alumni from 1962 to the present. The objective was to determine whether people with lower health risks, who tended to live longer than their peers, suffered greater disability (a decline in strength and increasing onset of debilitating diseases, for instance) as they grew older. In particular, the researchers evaluated the participants' smoking habits, weight levels, and exercise patterns.

They found that both men and women with high health risks—including smoking, obesity, or sedentary living—had twice the level of disability of those with low health risks. Also, the onset of disability was postponed by more than five years in the low-risk group, as compared with the high-risk group.

The researchers concluded that smoking habits, weight gains, and poor exercise patterns in midlife and late adulthood are predictors of subsequent disability. Furthermore, people with better health habits survive longer, the scientists said, and also, any disability they may experience is delayed and compressed into fewer years at the end of life. (See the *New England Journal of Medicine,* April 9, 1998; 338[15]: pp. 1035–41.)

This ability among fit, healthy older people to avoid disabilities by maintaining a high level of physical functioning almost until the time of death is what I've called in other contexts "squaring off the curve" of life. To understand how this works, it's helpful to think in terms of a line graph.

The lives of those people who fail to maintain good health habits would be plotted with a downward-curving graph line as they grow older. This line would represent their steady deterioration of physical abilities—such as loss of steadiness and stamina in walking, decline in strength levels, and increasing onset of debilitating diseases.

In contrast, the graph for older people who avoid smoking, who keep their weight within a healthy range, and who exercise regularly could be pictured as a squared-off line. In other words, the graph line that represents their ability to function effectively as they age remains high until some point near the end of life. Then, it plunges close to the time of death, as their final illness overtakes them. This kind of vigorous independence, which lasts until the final year or so of existence, is what we should all shoot for as we pursue our quest for that special vigor and personal energy, which define the power of youth.

Now, to give you a more complete set of tools for "squaring off the curve" in your life, let's turn to some specific concerns for your age-group—the immediate "pre-boomer," "boomer" and "post-boomer" generations, from about age thirty to the early seventies.

Part 2

....

The Ages of Target Training

7
. . . .

The Race Is to the Swift:
The Boomer Years and Beyond

The term *baby boomer,* or *boomer* for short, has come to refer specifically to those men and women born from 1946 to 1964. As this book is published, the category encompasses people who are about thirty-five to fifty-three years of age—and this is the group I'm highlighting in this chapter.

But in fact, much of what is contained here will apply to those who are a few years younger, and certainly to many who are considerably older—even as old as sixty-five to seventy-five. The key issue is not what your chronological age is, but rather, how old you are biologically and emotionally.

My main objective here, as well as elsewhere in this book, is to encourage you to begin wherever you are—and then to devise and follow a realistic plan for becoming younger. There is no single technique, supplement, or diet that will help you regain the power of youth—no magic bullet or special fountain of youth. Rather, recovering the energy and vigor you have lost is a step-by-step process. It's a matter of keying in on your weaknesses—"targeting" them, if you will—and then selecting responses that will provide you with that part of your youthful power that you have lost.

What are the most important challenges to youthful health and energy that the "boomers-and-beyond" generation should prepare to meet and overcome?

Turn Back the Clock

First and foremost, remember the basic targeting trilogy: strike, strengthen, and stretch. Be sure that you set up a regular fitness regimen, with strength work and endurance work balanced according to your age, as explained in Chapter 2 (i.e., the older you are, the more you need to weight your program toward strength training).

Also, be sure to include some "striking" or impact exercise to build up your bones. Obviously, this component of a fitness program has to be monitored carefully so as to avoid joint and muscle injury. But remember: as you move beyond about age thirty, your muscle and bone mass decline regularly with age. You can slow or even stop this process with a wisely targeted fitness program.

Finally, flexibility becomes increasingly important as you grow older. While you may have gotten away with stretching two or three times a week when you were younger, you'll most likely find you need to plug in a daily round of stretches as you move into your forties, and certainly your fifties.

Here's an outline of further targeting measures I would suggest to help turn back the clock:

- Target your health fears—and replace them with facts. Most likely, your health worries focus on issues that will never come to pass—yet you are probably overlooking and failing to prepare for health problems that are much more likely to strike you.
- Target your nutrition—and choose food that will empower and heal. In exploring this topic, we'll go into specific foods that will prepare you with staying power before you face a challenge, and

also those that will give you a quick surge of energy to help you recover after the challenge.

- Target your personal and family history—and learn to reduce your risks for certain diseases that may threaten you because of your background. If you have a family history of heart disease but no history of cancer, it stands to reason that you should make cardiovascular protection your main concern. We'll explore such considerations, including how you can deal with "good" and "bad" genes.
- Target your gender—and plan your health program according to the special risks you face because of your sex.
- Understand the latest diagnostic tools and treatments—and evaluate whether you should take advantage of them. In particular, we'll examine the benefits of the new fast CT scan and discuss whether it's worth it for you to lay out the money for one of these evaluations.
- Target your "outside" risks—and determine how you can reduce those risks. Accidents are one of the greatest causes of injuries and deaths—yet much of the risk could be lowered by taking certain simple precautions.
- Target your mind—and explore ways that you can maintain your mental acuity as you age.

These are the main issues we'll be discussing in this chapter, and these same themes will continue through the next two chapters, which deal first with the concerns of "young senior powerhouses," age seventy-six and older, and then with children, adolescents, and younger adults, up to about age thirty. But now, let's turn to our first "targeting" issue—the health fears and misconceptions that you may be harboring.

Target Your Health Fears

Replace your fears about your health with facts. The majority of American adults—53 percent—list cancer as the disease they most fear they might die from. Heart disease is a distant second, with only 37 percent of adults being afraid they might die of this condition. (*The Wall Street Journal*/NBC News poll, June 25, 1998.)

But the facts don't measure up to these fears.

Actually, more than sixty million Americans suffer from some kind of cardiovascular disease, such as blocked coronary arteries, high blood pressure, or stroke. Furthermore, nearly a million die each year from cardiovascular problems.

In contrast, only about eight million Americans have a history of cancer, and about a half million die each year from some form of cancer. Also, there's new hope here. Cancer rates began to decline in 1992, and deaths from cancer started to drop in 1996.

What do these trends suggest? Certainly, we shouldn't focus only on reducing our risks for heart disease and forget about cancer. But the cardiovascular threat should still be our first priority in preventive efforts, with cancer prevention a solid second.

Youth Booster
Aerobic Exercise: A Targeting Strategy for "Bad" Cholesterol?

In a July 2, 1998, study conducted at the Stanford University School of Medicine and published in the *New England Journal of Medicine* (Vol. 339, No. 1, pp. 12–20), researchers explored the effects of aerobic exercise on "bad" (low-density lipoprotein, or "LDL") cholesterol.

The participants included 180 postmenopausal women, ages forty-five to sixty-four, and 197 men, ages thirty through sixty-four. The subjects had moderately high levels of LDL cholesterol for their gender and age levels.

The participants were divided randomly into four groups: 1) those who did aerobic exercise only; 2) those on a diet established by the National Cholesterol Education Program (NCEP), which was moderately low in fat and cholesterol;

3) those who engaged in both exercise and the diet; and 4) a group consisting of controls who received no medical intervention.

The results showed that the diet by itself failed to lower the "bad" LDL cholesterol levels in men or women. But when combined with aerobic exercise, the diet did lower the LDL by an average of 20 mg/dl in the men, and more than 14 mg/dl in the women. The researchers concluded that physical activity is important in treating elevated LDL cholesterol.

The main message I'm trying to get across here is this: boomers should plan a preventive health program based on the facts, not on fantasies or unfounded fears. This means taking into account the actual statistical health risks you face, and then balancing these numbers against your particular personal and family health history.

Obviously, statistics relating to the general population aren't the controlling factor if you have a particular health problem. For example, you may be one of the twenty-one million Americans who suffer regularly from heartburn. If so, you may be able to handle the condition by adjusting your diet so as to reduce or eliminate offending foods (e.g., especially spicy dishes, caffeine, alcohol, chocolate, or just overeating), or by taking common antacids such as Tums, Mylanta, Tagamet, or Maalox.

On the other hand, the heartburn may be a sign of a more persistent disorder, which requires targeting strategies directed by a physician. A tip-off that you may be suffering from something more than garden-variety heartburn or indigestion is that no matter how many antacids you take, you get no relief.

In such a case, the problem may be a medical condition such as gastroesophageal reflux disease, or GERD. This is potentially a serious, but still treatable medical problem, which researchers estimate may trouble up to 10 percent of adult Americans. It's important to get medical treatment for GERD as early as possible because the condition can lead to stomach ulcers or inflammation of the esophagus. There may also be more serious complications, such as cancer of the esophagus—which, incidentally, is one of the few cancers still on the rise in the United States.

Symptoms to watch for include frequent heartburn (two or more times a week, especially at night); a lingering, sour taste; constant need for antacids and excessive belching. Also, you may have difficulty swallowing food and experience hoarseness or coughing. In many cases, the condition becomes worse when you lie down.

Fortunately, a qualified physician can usually treat GERD successfully with prescription drugs and specific dietary changes. But it's important for you, the patient, to notify your doctor about your symptoms and get his "targeted" medical help as soon as possible. The longer you wait, the greater your risk of serious complications.

I mention this problem of heartburn just to put any fears you may have in perspective. Certainly, it's important to survey your overall risk of heart disease, cancer, and other high-profile illnesses and to organize your fitness and preventive health regimen accordingly.

But it's even more important to focus on any personal history you may have of cancer or diabetes—or serious heartburn. Similarly, you should take special note if you've had a parent under age fifty or fifty-five who died of a cardiovascular problem. These are particular factors that you should place a priority on when you're designing your personal health program. Such facts about your life and background are always more important than the fears you may feel after watching a TV report about some particularly horrendous disease—which you are highly unlikely to get. (For more on this issue, see "Target Your Personal and Family History" on page 210.)

The following box will give you an idea of just how beneficial a personal health program can be.

Rx Response
A Targeting Treatment Does Double Duty for Hypertension and Diabetes

As the "Father of Aerobics," I may be expected to have a certain bias in favor of endurance exercise. But I'm constantly amazed at how study after study seems to confirm a panacea-like effect for this sort of activity. Two recent studies are cases in point.

The December 1997 issue of *Circulation* reported that even one week of daily aerobic exercise can reduce the risks of diabetes by improving the body's sensitivity to insulin. In this University of Pittsburgh study, eleven overweight, inactive African-American women, who had "insulin resistance" that could lead to diabetes, aerobic exercise increased their insulin sensitivity by an average of 58 percent. Five of the women were no longer insulin resistant at all. Also, their fasting insulin levels fell by 20 percent—a sign that their risks for diabetes had dropped markedly.

In another study on hypertension among African-American men, researchers from the Veterans Affairs Medical Center in Washington, D.C., confirmed that moderate endurance exercise can significantly lower blood pressure. The study, published on November 30, 1995, in the *New England Journal of Medicine,* involved forty-six men with blood pressure higher than 180 (systolic) over 110 (diastolic).

Their pressure was first brought under control with medications, and then the men were placed on a regimen of sixteen weeks of endurance exercise on stationary cycles. They rode forty-five minutes per day at 75 percent of their maximum heart rate. After sixteen weeks, their lower, or diastolic, number fell from 88 to 83, while the pressure of a nonexercising control group went up. After another sixteen weeks of exercise, the cyclers were able to lower their hypertension drugs by 30 to 40 percent. (See *The New York Times,* Nov. 30, 1995, p. A16.)

Caution: Although aerobic exercise may be a great targeting strategy for both diabetes and hypertension, those with these serious conditions should always consult their physicians and undergo a thorough medical exam, including a stress test, before they embark on such a regimen. Also, with high blood pressure, heavy resistance exercise, such as intensive weight lifting, should be avoided.

Before we leave this issue of serious diseases—and the fears often associated with them—let me suggest one final word of caution about the limits of the targeting strategy, as I have advocated it in this book. Many of the conditions we've been discussing in these pages, such as mild aches, pains, and fatigue, can be handled through a self-treatment response.

But when you move into the area of heart disease, cancer, diabetes, and the like, it's absolutely essential that you avoid self-treatment!

Failing to seek professional medical help for a nagging problem like the serious heartburn situation described earlier may lead to disaster. In any case, delay will usually result in additional complications, which could have been avoided by consulting a physician at an early stage.

Even with the most serious health conditions, however, targeting can still play a role. Targeting, remember, involves self-assessment, as well as self-treatment. The wise patient should always be checking his own physical and emotional condition. Such a vigilant, alert stance will, in turn, be more likely to cause him to see the doctor at an early date—and enhance the possibility of an effective doctor-patient collaboration during treatment. (The Cooper Energy Scale in Chapter 3 is specifically designed to work well for this sort of self-assessment prior to a visit to a physician.)

By remaining alert and sensitive to your body's responses, then, you'll be much more likely to remain rooted in the facts and less likely to fall prey to any unfounded fears associated with your health. For a practical illustration showing why relying on your doctor, rather than on yourself is essential for hypertension management, read the following box.

Rx Response
Where Physicians Must Supervise a Targeting Strategy:Lowering Blood Pressure to Reduce Heart Attack Risk

Too often, patients with high blood pressure think they can decide on their own about when to take their medications. In some cases, these patients become frustrated because of the reduction in sexual performance that accompanies some drugs. Others fool themselves into believing that so long as they stay below the commonly accepted minimum of 140/90, they are safe.

A new set of studies, reported at a meeting of the International Society for Hypertension in Amsterdam on June 10, 1998, shows that such attitudes are not only wrong—they may also be dangerous. One report, the Hypertension Optimal Treatment study, involving more than eighteen thousand patients who were followed for an average of four years, showed that using drugs to lower the diastolic (lower) blood pressure number from 90 to 80 could reduce the incidence of heart attacks by 37 percent.

In another part of the study, researchers found that the ACE inhibitor Captopril (Capoten, Capozide) was more effective than diuretics and beta-blockers in reducing the incidence of heart attacks and strokes, including the risk of death. (See *The Wall Street Journal,* June 10, 1998, p. B10.)

Target Your Nutrition

Many of the "boomers" I have encountered seem obsessed with food—but they appear to know little about how to use it to enhance their health and energize their bodies and minds.

I constantly have to respond to people who are wondering about new, faddish diets—such as those that include inordinate amounts of protein or fat, or are otherwise unbalanced. Yet when you come down to it, designing a good, basic food plan is rather simple. I've mentioned the major elements of a good diet in Chapter 6—such as the importance of:

- fiber and cruciferous vegetables
- the need to reduce intake of saturated and "trans" (hydrogenated, or hardened) fats
- the minimum intake of fluids—and the importance of avoiding "negative" drinks, such as those containing caffeine and alcohol, which act as diuretics to draw fluids from your body
- the need to strike the right balance among carbohydrates, protein, and fats
- my recommended dosages of such essential antioxidants and other supplements as vitamin E, vitamin C, and folic acid

But there is another set of issues I want to mention at this point—the use of food to manage your energy needs from day to day, and activity to activity. When you're considering your energy requirements, it's helpful to distinguish between nutritional responses and targeting strategies for two different situations:

- a demanding event that you are on the verge of facing—whether a high-stress effort at work or a potentially exhausting athletic event or workout; and
- a demanding, draining event that you have already faced

In the first situation, you need to build up your stores of energy; in the second, you need to replenish them. These two differing demands require different nutritional strategies, though both should be based on a concept known as the "glycemic index."

This term refers to the ranking of foods not according to their basic nutritional value, but according to the degree to which they trigger blood glucose (sugar) and insulin responses. In general, foods that are low on the glycemic index—i.e., those that cause a relatively slow increase in blood sugar and insulin—should be consumed before a demanding event because research has shown that they increase energy, endurance, and overall muscular and cardiovascular staying power. In contrast, foods that are high on the glycemic index should be eaten after a demanding event because they feed into the bloodstream more quickly, replenish muscle glycogen (sugars), and restore any energy you may have lost.

Now, let's look at some foods that you can select for each energy pack targeting strategy—preparing for a demanding event, or recovering from such an event. (Sources include "International tables of glycemic index," by Kaye Foster-Powell and Janette Brand Miller, *American Journal of Clinical Nutrition,* 1995; 62: pp. 871S–93S.)

Nutritional Targeting Strategy #1:
Preparing for a Demanding Event

Consider this sampling of foods that are relatively low on the glycemic index, and thus should supply you with the energy you need to maintain endurance during a demanding athletic, occupational, or other personal challenge:

barley kernel bread (50 percent or more kernels)
oat bran bread (45 percent or more oat bran)
rye kernel bread (80 percent kernels)
pumpernickel bread
All-Bran cereal
skim milk (excellent)
low-fat yogurt (excellent)
apples, whole (excellent)

grapefruit, whole (excellent)
oranges, whole (good)
pears, whole (good)
dried beans (excellent)
chickpeas (excellent)
kidney beans (excellent)
lentils (excellent)
soya beans (excellent)
pasta (e.g., fettuccini, linguine) (good)
spaghetti (excellent)

sweet potatoes

yams

lentil soup

fructose sugars (excellent)

lactose (milk) sugars

dried peas (excellent)

green peas

Nutritional Targeting Strategy #2:
Recovering from a Demanding Event

Here are some illustrations of foods that are high on the glycemic index, and thus appropriate for use in a targeting strategy designed to pick you up and infuse you with energy you have just lost:

angel food cake

croissant

doughnut, cake-type

corn muffins

bran muffins

waffles

bagel

white bread

whole wheat or whole-meal
   bread

Cheerios cereal

corn flakes

Cream of Wheat cereal

Grape Nuts Flakes

Rice Krispies cereal

Shredded Wheat cereal

Total cereal

instant rice

most crackers

carrots

baked potatoes

honey

Once again, remember that selecting foods according to where they stand on the glycemic index has nothing to do with their basic nutritional value. In other words, carrots, baked potatoes, and many types of bagels are excellent foods in the sense that they provide many nutrients that our bodies need. But it's best to eat them after a demanding, energy-sapping challenge rather than before the event. The reason: they are low on the glycemic index and feed quickly into your bloodstream. That's a good quality if you want a quick surge of energy, but not if you want stores of energy that have to last over a period of hours. So when you want to use nutrition as part of a targeting strategy to hike your energy levels, it's essential to take the glycemic index into account.

For more on the energy benefits of the bagel, see the accompanying box.

Energy Pack
Tapping the Power of a Bagel

One of the items listed among the "high" glycemic index foods in the accompanying text is the bagel. In other words, this bread product, like others in the "high" category, has the power to infuse you with energy after an exhausting bout of exercise—but how does this idea work out in practice?

Researchers from Ball State University reported in January 1988 on their research on the ability of bagels, versus commercial energy bars, to help competitive bicyclists recover from a rigorous series of rides. After becoming thoroughly fatigued, the riders were given either the energy bars or bagels as pick-me-up snacks. Six hours later, they were put back on their bicycles and rode at their own pace for an additional hour.

The researchers found that the bagels did as good a job as the energy bars in providing the athletes with energy to perform work and use their respiratory systems. The manufacturers of the energy bars noted that their products provided extra nutrients, such as vitamin C and iron. But the investigators emphasized that the bagels provided the same energy benefits as the bars. (See report in *The Washington Post,* reprinted in *The Palm Beach Post,* Jan. 24, 1998, p. 5D.)

Another important targeting feature related to nutrition is weight control. In Chapter 6, we've already discussed some of the important issues related to obesity, including excess weight as an independent risk factor for various diseases. But there are a couple of other points that must be made—one that is well known, and another that may be rather surprising.

First, the well-known point: if you want to lose or gain weight, you must become aware of your caloric intake. I know this isn't a particularly exciting idea. Many people would rather look for unusual new "miracle" diets that they think will allow them to run around the calorie issue. But in the end, if you want to lose weight and keep it off, you must take in fewer calories than you expend—and also combine your reduced food intake with an increase in aerobic and strength exercise. (For more details, see the discussion on this issue in Chapter 6.)

But now consider a more surprising point: exercise may make more of a difference in your weight-loss efforts than you've been led to expect. In fact, it may even be possible for you to devise fitness strategies to target certain parts of your body for spot reduction.

The common wisdom in the medical community has usually been that such attempts at spot reduction don't work. In other words, if you have excess fat on your thighs or around your middle, the only way you can get rid of it is to go on a general weight-loss program. Then, as you lose weight all over your body, you'll also get rid of a proportionate amount in the areas that most concern you.

Certainly, a general weight-loss program must be the cornerstone of any weight-loss effort, regardless of your specific objectives. If you lose overall weight by cutting down on your calorie intake, you'll also take off some fat on your stomach, thighs, and bottom.

But there are also some studies suggesting that, in addition to adjusting your diet, you can successfully target particular fatty areas with specific types of exercise. Here is the evidence as it stands at this writing:

Strength training resulted in significant reductions in "intra-abdominal adipose tissue," or fatty tissue deep inside the abdomen, according to an April 1995 report in the *Journal of Applied Physiology* (Vol. 78, No. 4, pp. 1425–31).

The fourteen participants, with a mean age of sixty-seven, engaged in total-body strength training three times per week for sixteen weeks. Their training intensity was gradually increased so that they were working out with resistance equal to about 67 percent of what they could lift with one repetition.

Although they experienced no significant changes in total body weight or total body fat, they did shift the arrangement of their fat: they lost significant amounts of intra-abdominal fat and also fat tissue just beneath the skin on their midthigh region. Also, they significantly increased their upper body strength by 51 percent, and their lower body strength by 65 percent.

An April 1998 study in *Scandinavian Journal of Medical Science and Sports* (Vol. 8, No. 2, pp. 102–8) focused on the body composition of 120 men—including twenty-two elite runners, eighty-six recreational runners, and twelve nonrunning controls.

The researchers determined that when compared with the controls, the fat percentage in the abdominal area of the long-distance runners was 42 percent lower, and the fat in the thighs was 36 percent lower. Also, they determined that the fat percentages were associated with the training intensity. (The more you run, the lower the fat percentage in those two areas.) In addition, the testosterone levels contributed strongly to the fat percentage in the abdominal region.

Although women generally lose weight less easily than men in response to exercise, intensive endurance exercise can have an effect—especially on abdominal fat.

That was the conclusion of an August 1991, fourteen-month study published in the *American Journal of Physiology* (Vol. 261, No. 2, Part 1, pp. E159–67). In this investigation, thirteen obese premenopausal women, averaging almost thirty-nine years of age, exercised four to five times per week for ninety minutes at approximately 55 percent of their maximal aerobic power.

The researchers found that the exercisers experienced a significant increase in their aerobic power and reduction in their total body fat mass. Furthermore, they experienced a greater loss of abdominal fat versus midthigh fat.

These and related studies suggest that a kind of spot reduction is possible—if you engage in intensive exercise. High doses of strength and endurance training seem to work well in reducing both thigh and abdominal fat in men. Women, whose bodies are more resistant to the fat-reduction powers of exercise, seem to do better in their stomach and thigh weight-loss efforts with aerobic exercises, such as running. With both men and women, however, it's important not to forget calorie restriction: a nutritional targeting strategy that focuses only on exercise—whether the purpose is general weight loss or spot reduction—will almost always fail unless you cut your calories as well.

Target Your Personal and Family History

One of the most important phases of the total physical exams we conduct at the Cooper Clinic is the personal and family health history that our patients fill out. In many respects, this is a rough evaluation of the state of your genes—what qualities you've inherited from your parents or grandparents that raise or lower your risks of certain health problems.

There is almost always a genetic or inherited factor at work in all the major diseases—including cancer, diabetes, and cardiovascular problems, such as the "hardening of the arteries" (atherosclerosis) that leads to heart attacks, stroke, and high blood pressure.

Obviously, there's nothing you can do to change these "givens" in your inheritance. But you can often reduce their impact by concentrating hard on lowering other risk factors.

One of the best examples of how this works is with heart disease. If you have a parent who died of a heart attack at age fifty or younger, your risks are much higher than a person with both parents still living at the ripe old age of ninety.

What can you do to counter these "bad genes" in your background? Our usual recommendation, which is backed up by considerable scientific evidence, is that you should work harder than most people to lower your other cardiovascular risks factors—such as high cholesterol, high blood pressure, smoking, obesity, sedentary living, and the like.

Take a situation confronted by my wife, Millie. Several years ago, she had an abnormal stress test, and I thought it had to be a "false positive"—in short, a mistake—because of her low-risk profile for cardiovascular disease. She was a regular runner, had a healthy lipid and cholesterol range, wasn't obese, and in general, seemed quite healthy.

But when she returned for a second test a couple of years later, the results were even worse. So we ordered a stress echocardiogram to check her heart even more thoroughly.

Although this result also signaled possible problems, I refused to believe she had coronary disease. So I told her to try still another stress test. This one came back with the worst result yet.

"Just to prove that these tests are all false positives, we'll do an ultrafast CT scan," I announced, and Millie, good sport that she is, agreed.

This highly sophisticated evaluation involved having a picture taken of her heart and other upper-body organs with a new diagnostic device. This scan, which involves an eight-minute procedure using electrodes and computerized imaging, is proving to be a great way to identify calcification (blockage with plaque) of the coronary arteries, tumors, and other internal diseases.

This time, the results were definitive. Millie's calcification score of 763 was off the chart, putting her in the top (worst) percentile for her age-group.

But we still didn't have the answer to what was causing her problem. Knowing that her cholesterol tests had presented us with a dead end, I turned to the new homocysteine test, which many feel is now becoming as important for detecting cardiovascular risk as the cholesterol checkup.

This time, we struck pay dirt. Her homocysteine score was 21—a level that placed her far up in the highest risk category.

Fortunately, there was a clear and powerful response to this problem: folic acid. Millie began to take 800 mcg of folic acid daily through our Cooper Complete nutritional supplement program. Within eight weeks, her homocysteine levels were down to 8.0, or the low-risk category.

An interesting genetic twist to Millie's problem is that we found that her mother's homocysteine count was also 21, and the older woman had already suffered several heart attacks. Predictably, the mother's calcification score was even higher than Millie's.

On the other hand, Millie's older sister, Alice, was the beneficiary of an entirely different line of inherited genes. Her homocysteine level, without taking any folic acid or any other special steps to lower her other cardiovascular risk factors, was only 9.0. Also, her coronary vessel calcification score was only 43—or about what you'd expect for a woman in her thirties, not sixties.

"It's not fair," Millie said. "I've tried to do everything right, and I'm the one with the vessel problem."

"It's the luck of the draw," I said. "You got your mother's genes, and Alice inherited your father's."

Millie's father lived to age eighty-five and died of cancer—but didn't have a trace of coronary artery disease.

Also, having a mother, sister, or both who have suffered from breast cancer greatly increases your risks of the same disease. But that's no reason to become deterministic and decide it's inevitable that you'll get the disease as well.

Instead, you should be particularly alert to doing self-exams of your breasts, and don't delay if you notice any changes in the breast structure or the appearance of a suspicious lump or nodule. Most likely, your relative who suffered from the disease didn't act as quickly as she should have in seeking medical help. Frequent mammograms—at least every other year after age forty and annually after age fifty—are also essential. In addition, there are many other preventive steps you can take, including lowering the intake of fat in your diet.

In some areas, we're moving quickly beyond these rough measures of risk toward a more precise determination of exactly what your genetic weaknesses and strengths may be. Here are a few illustrations:

Cancer

The discovery of a brain cancer gene, P-Ten, has opened the door to diagnosing and treating a fatal form of brain cancer that kills most of its fifteen thousand American victims each year. (See the March 28, 1997 issue of *Science,* reported in *The Wall Street Journal,* March 28, 1997, p. B2.)

An estrogen gene, CYP17—which is carried by 40 percent of women and may double their risk and be responsible for 30 percent of all breast cancer cases—has been discovered by scientists from the University of Southern California. (From a report at a conference of the American Cancer Society, published March 25, 1997.)

Alzheimer's Disease

Alzheimer's disease has been linked to a protein produced by a gene known as apolipoprotein E ("apo E"). People with a particular version of these gene, apo E-2, are four times as likely to live long lives as those with another variation, apo E-4. Also, those with apo E-2 are much less likely to develop Alzheimer's at an early age than those with apo E-4. In addition, research has shown that men and women with the "bad" apo E-4 gene are more likely to develop coronary heart disease.

What use is this knowledge? For one thing, researchers expect that soon they will be able to use it to make an early diagnosis for Alzheimer's. In the longer term, scientists are working with drugmakers to develop a drug that provides the same protection that the apo E-2 gene does. (See *The Wall Street Journal,* Oct. 19, 1995, p. 1.)

Osteoporosis

Osteoporosis has been connected to a gene known as COLIA1, according to the *New England Journal of Medicine* (April 9, 1998; 338: pp. 1016–21).

Those with variations of this gene may inherit either high or low bone density. Other studies of twins have established that about 80 percent of variations in bone mass at different ages can be accounted for by genetic factors.

So what do you do if you find you have this gene?

A *NEJM* editorial accompanying the above report notes that there is a great deal of evidence showing that relatives of patients with osteoporosis have a high probability of having low bone density—a major risk factor for the disease—and that includes relatives with no symptoms. So members of these families should consider having their bone mineral density measured regularly. If the results are abnormal, they may need to change their approach to diet and exercise, and perhaps even embark on drug therapy before the loss of bone becomes extensive or irreversible.

These examples provide you with an idea of the rate at which gene research is progressing. Such efforts as the Human Genome Project, sponsored by the National Institutes of Health and the Department of Energy, are moving toward a complete mapping of human genetic structure by the year 2005 at a cost of $3 billion. Once the genes that cause specific diseases are identified, scientists will be in a position to take the next step—developing means to diagnose and treat the conditions. It's definitely to your advantage to keep abreast of these breakthroughs.

So if you think you've found some information about this gene research that may affect you or your family, don't hesitate to ask your physician about the prospects for a targeted solution, such as drugs or other treatments. Many times, patients who take the initiative are the first to find a life-saving response to a health threat.

Target Your Gender

It may seem silly to say, in effect, "when considering your health, note whether you are a man or a woman." But this is one of those obvious points that is often overlooked, even by physicians and scientists.

One of the great medical omissions in recent years has been the failure to do a sufficient number of studies on women for such problems as heart disease. Because women were largely protected from this disease until menopause, most of the focus has been on men, and especially middle-aged men.

But now, with many more women living for decades past

menopause, more are dying from cardiovascular disease because, having passed through menopause, they lack the protection from estrogen that they had in their younger days. As a result, an increasing number of studies are being done on the heart, stroke, and other vessel disease risks facing older women. Also, treatments are being adjusted to accommodate these risks.

For example, consider the issue of hormone replacement therapy (HRT), which is often prescribed for women who have moved through menopause. Should you undergo this therapy, or shouldn't you?

A *JAMA* study reported on August 19, 1998, by University of California researchers determined that women with heart disease should avoid HRT after menopause. The investigators said that women with heart disease faced a 50 percent higher risk of a heart attack than patients who were placed on placebos. (See *USA Today*, Aug. 19, 1998, p. 1.)

The answer also depends on your specific health risks for heart disease, osteoporosis, breast cancer, and a number of other conditions. For more details, see the accompanying chart that provides an overview and action guide for five typical women going through menopause.

Targeting Five Postmenopausal Women:
The Cooper Recommendations for
Hormone Replacement Therapy (HRT)

Woman #1:
Three or more of these coronary risk factors:

- Family history of heart disease
- Elevated cholesterol
- Hypertension (high blood pressure)
- Cigarette smoking
- Sedentary lifestyle
- Diabetes

Targeting response, if she is willing to change all possible risk factors:

- No hormone replacement therapy (HRT)
- Aggressive risk factor modification (i.e., cholesterol control, lower hypertension, stop cigarette smoking, begin regular exercise program, control of diabetes)
- Possible lipid-lowering drugs
- Vitamin E (>400 IU/day)
- Calcium (1,500 mg/day), with vitamin D (600 IU/day)
- Weight-bearing, impact exercise
- Aspirin (81 mg/day)

Targeting response, if she won't change risk factors:

- Hormone replacement therapy (HRT)
- Vitamin E (>400 IU/day)
- Calcium (1,500 mg/day), with vitamin D (600 IU/day)
- Aspirin (81 mg/day)

Woman #2:
Known personal history of osteoporosis or bone loss

Targeting response:

- Hormone replacement therapy (HRT)
- Aggressive risk factor modification
- Vitamin E (>400 IU/day)
- Calcium (1,500 mg/day), with vitamin D (600 IU/day)
- Weight-bearing, impact ("striking") exercise
- Aspirin (81 mg/day)

Woman# 3:
Known personal history or strong family history of breast cancer, with or without coronary risk factors

Targeting response:

- No hormone replacement therapy (HRT)
- Aggressive risk factor modification (i.e., cholesterol control, lower hypertension, stop cigarette smoking, begin regular exercise program, control of diabetes)
- Possible lipid-lowering drugs
- Vitamin E (>400 IU/day)
- Calcium (1,500 mg/day), with vitamin D (600 IU/day)
- Weight-bearing, impact ("striking") exercise
- Aspirin (81 mg/day)

Woman #4:
No coronary risk factors, no memopausal symptoms, and normal bone density

Targeting response:

- No hormone replacement therapy (HRT)
- Vitamin E (>400 IU/day)
- Calcium (1,500 mg/day), with vitamin D (600 IU/day)
- Weight-bearing, impact ("striking") exercise
- Reevaluate risk annually

Woman #5:
Severe problems with menopausal symptoms, such as:

- Vasomotor symptoms (hot flushes, etc.)
- Fatigue
- Memory or concentration problems
- Headaches
- Decreased libido
- Mood disturbances (such as depression)

Targeting response:

- Phytoestrogens (weak estrogens contained in certain foods, such as soy products or wild yams)
- Evening primrose oil
- Other herbal treatments (See the "Hormone" and "Herbs" entries in my *Advanced Nutritional Therapies.*)
- If no improvement, use hormone replacement therapy (HRT) unless there is a personal history of heart disease or breast cancer.

I've already introduced many of the other health concerns and biological changes that occur in women during menopause in the youth drain discussion in Chapter 4. Also, at that point we explored the differences between traditional female menopause and "male menopause," an extended period of change for men that involves many hormonal and physical transformations.

But here are just a few more distinctives that make women emotionally and biologically special. An understanding of these can help you adjust your expectations—and in many cases, prepare yourself in ways that may help preserve the power of youth.

Sensitivity to Pain

Women may be more sensitive to pain than men. At a conference on gender and pain sponsored by the National Institutes of Health in April 1998, several experts suggested that women perceive and react more quickly than men to biological signals that something may be wrong.

There isn't agreement about whether women actually feel pain more than men, or whether they have been conditioned to react more quickly. But some scientists believe that the female hormone estrogen may sensitize women to pain more than men.

According to one report at the conference, Ohio University studies on people suffering from osteoarthritis have shown that women are more likely than men to rely on pain-management techniques, such as relaxation strategies or seeking sympathy and help from others. Other studies done at the Harvard Medical School on pain following injuries to nerves have shown that these pains tend to occur five times more in girls than in boys.

Muscular Pain and Weakness

Many women in early middle age experience aches, weaknesses, and an inability to perform simple daily tasks. In a federally financed study, the Study of Women Across America, which is being conducted by the University of Michigan's School of Public Health, preliminary findings released on October 14, 1997, revealed that middle-aged women feel more pain and are weaker than many experts expected.

Among the ten thousand women in the study, who ranged from age forty to fifty-five, 8 percent reported that they had significant difficulty climbing a flight of stairs, carrying groceries, or even walking around the block. A surprising 20 percent said they had some difficulty performing these actions.

Also, 55 percent of the women said that in the past two weeks, they had suffered from soreness or stiffness in their necks, backs, or shoulders.

Fear of Breast Cancer

Most older women fear breast cancer so much that they fail to protect themselves against heart attacks—which pose a bigger threat. A survey by the National Council on the Aging, which was released on November 18, 1997, focused on the fear of disease among more than one thousand women, ages forty-five to fifty-four. More than half, or 61 percent, said they were most afraid of all types of cancer—but only 9 percent said they feared a heart attack. Yet heart attacks are the number one killer of American females. (About 50 percent of all women will die from cardiovascular disease.)

About 24 percent of these women said they were most worried about breast cancer, versus 7 percent who named lung cancer. Yet lung cancer is the biggest cancer threat among women.

Medication for Depression

Depressed women typically respond better to different drugs from those that work on men. A 1998 report in the *Journal of Clinical Psychiatry* said that depressed men appear to respond most readily to medications that affect two neurotransmitter networks—norepinephrine and serotonin. But women respond better to drugs that influence the serotonin only. (See *The New York Times,* June 21, 1998, Sec. 15, p.1.)

Risk of Cervical Cancer

Unfaithful husbands may give their wives cervical cancer. In a study published in the August 7, 1996, issue of the *Journal of the National Cancer Institute,* researchers from the Johns Hopkins University School of Medicine reported that promiscuous male sexual behavior is a key factor in cervical cancer.

They said that women are five to eleven times as likely to get cervical cancer if their male partners have had sex with prostitutes or multiple women. This particular cancer is linked to a virus that is spread by sexual intercourse.

But there is another side to this coin: women can turn the tables on themselves and put themselves at increased risk if they engage in sex with multiple partners.

Although these are some of the most recently reported findings that apply specifically to women, new information seems to come out almost every day. To keep up with the avalanche of new facts and recommendations—and avoid the possibility of confusion that may arise with conflicting accounts—refer back to the guidelines suggested in Chapter 6 on cutting through the medical confusion.

UNDERSTAND THE LATEST DIAGNOSTIC TOOLS AND TREATMENTS

It's impossible for busy, practicing physicians to keep track of all the latest scientific findings, medical procedures, drugs, and diagnostic machines—especially when this information isn't directly related to their specialty or practice.

For this reason, it's important for you to be thoroughly acquainted with your own individual set of risk factors, genetic predisposition, and personal and family health history. With this knowledge at your fingertips, you'll be much more likely to be alert to new developments that may have a direct effect on your health.

Obviously, you'll often hear about a new concept or procedure and think it relates directly to you, when really, it doesn't. But that's part of the reason you have enlisted the services of a personal physician: he is there not only to treat your immediate ailments and illnesses, but also to advise you about how new treatments or preventive measures may apply to your situation.

Here's an example of what I'm talking about. About four years ago while I was on a work-vacation stay at our vacation home in Colorado, I attended a social gathering, where I heard an amazing, too-good-to-be-true story. According to the report, a company by the name of Imatron had produced an amazing fast scanning machine— the Ultrafast CT scanner—that was supposed to be able to provide a highly accurate picture of the internal organs, heart, and vessels in only about eight to ten minutes.

I filed the information at the back of my mind—until some physicians rented a space from the Cooper Clinic in Dallas for the express purpose of offering exams using this Ultrafast CT scanner. One thing led to another, and now we at the Clinic are involved in doing our own tests—with great results. We've identified many blockages in coronary arteries, as well as tumors on various organs, such as the kidney and liver.

I tell this story for one major reason: even such a dramatic advance in screening for cardiovascular disease as this often emerges very slowly into the public consciousness.

Even though I am more aware of breakthroughs in diagnostic screening than most physicians, I was definitely not the first to hear about this device. Now, we have been using this technique with great success over the past couple of years, but still, the general public is almost totally unaware of the machine.

This may seem remarkable since a number of studies establishing the scanner's effectiveness have appeared in many major professional journals (e.g., *Circulation, JAMA,* and other publications). For that matter, the technique has been covered by *The Wall Street Journal,* the NBC *Today Show* and the *Nightly News* with Tom Brokaw.

So with all the publicity, why hasn't the word gotten out?

For one thing, there are still relatively few of the scanners in operation. They are quite expensive, costing several million dollars, and many medical institutions and hospitals have chosen not to lay out the money. Also, most physicians still seem to be unaware of the existence of the technique. Finally, the individual tests can be expensive, running as high as six hundred dollars. But in the near future, you'll be hearing much more about this technique, and many readers will actually undergo the tests.

Of course, this is only one example of the tremendous strides we'll be making soon in diagnosis and treatment of cardiovascular disease and many other serious illnesses. The challenge for you, the patient, is to be alert as medical news reports break, keep news clippings or printouts on those that seem to affect you—and if you find they do have some relevance to your health, develop a targeting strategy to make use of them.

Target "Outside" Risks

Too often in popular health books we focus exclusively on diseases (or problems "inside" our bodies) and completely forget about "outside" risks—especially the accidents that take so many lives each year. It's at least as important to target these dangers—and develop strategies to do something about them.

Here are some areas of particular concern:

- Job-related injuries and job-caused illnesses. In 1992 about 6,500 Americans died from work-related causes, and 13.2 million were injured on the job, according to research done at San Jose State University in California. Job-related factors resulted in such problems as lung disease and lead poisoning, which caused more than 60,000 deaths and 800,000 illnesses in 1992, according to the study. (See *The Wall Street Journal,* July 28, 1997, p. B9.)

- Motor vehicle fatalities and injuries. There were more than 44,000 road fatalities in 1996, with speed-associated crashes accounting for almost 31 percent of the total. In 1992 the number of fatalities was 42,000—and there were more than 2 million disabling injuries from vehicle accidents. About 45 percent of all traffic fatalities in 1992 involved some form of drunkenness. The "targeting" messages here are obvious: when you drive, avoid alcohol, don't speed—and buckle up.
- Firearm-related deaths. After traffic related deaths, firearms are the second leading cause of accidental death in the United States. In 1991, for instance, there were a total of more than 38,000 deaths from firearms.
- Home accidents. In 1993 there were 22,500 deaths from accidents around the home, including such factors as falls, poison, fire, and suffocation from swallowing an object.

I bring these matters to your attention not in an attempt to provide an exhaustive list, but just to encourage you to do some thinking. When you are trying to develop a targeting strategy to protect your own health and that of your family, it doesn't make sense to focus only on disease and to forget the obvious dangers and risks around the home, on the road, or at work. Targeting is more than a mere self-help medical concept. Rather, it's a lifestyle that features intelligent risk reduction and "treatments" that may have a medical component—but may also involve just plain old common sense.

Target Your Mind

One of the fears I encounter most often in my patients who are growing older is the fear of losing mental sharpness. There is the worry that memory will fade, that the ability to process information will decline, and that eventually dementia or Alzheimer's may take over.

It's true that certain types of mental processing do tend to decline with age, such as "elastic" thinking, or the ability to process new information as quickly as we could when we were quite young. On the other hand, for those who stay fit and in good health, any loss of speed is usually more than made up for by the increased wisdom and greater accumulation of knowledge that accompanies aging.

What are some of the major strategies you should consider for keeping up your mental keenness as you age? Here are a few that have worked for me and for others as well:

Stay Optimistic

In another context, we explored how pessimism can sap your vigor and energy and make you old before your time. It can affect your mind and body negatively as well.

On a purely practical level, I find that assuming a "can-do" attitude about my work or personal aspirations always opens up possibilities. My mind begins to work in new, creative ways—and I'm sure that, physiologically, the neurotransmitters in my brain are finding new pathways and enhancing the overall thinking process. Optimism helps me focus and concentrate better—and that automatically gives me a more vigorous and youthful drive as I tackle new projects and ideas.

Direct health benefits also go along with optimism. In the June 1998 issue of the *Journal of Personality and Social Psychology,* for example, researchers from the University of Kentucky in Lexington reported on how positive or negative feelings could affect the immune systems of law students.

Those who were "situational optimists"—i.e., who had an upbeat, positive attitude when they were facing a challenge or crisis, such as an exam—had relatively strong immune systems. In fact, they found that one measurement of immunity, the levels of T-cells, rose by 13 percent when the situational optimists were facing a challenge, but dropped by 3 percent in situational pessimists.

What can you do if you are more of a pessimist than an optimist when you confront a difficult task? The researchers said that no one's pessimism is written in stone. You can learn to become more optimistic through techniques of cognitive therapy—such as pinpointing negative thoughts and then transforming them in your mind into a more positive form. (See *The New York Times,* June 30, 1998, p. B15.)

Develop Memory Techniques

Using "tricks" to remember lists is an old, proven technique that I've used all my life. And now that I'm pushing seventy, I find that some of these methods are as helpful as they've ever been.

For example, when I prepare for one of the hundreds of radio, TV, or newspaper interviews I do every year, I try to reduce important concepts to just a few memorable words, letters, or memorable pictures.

I might refer to the importance of eating cruciferous vegetables as nutritional protection against cancer, and inevitably a reporter will ask, "What are those vegetables?"

It's easy to draw a blank at such a question, regardless of your age—unless you have a trick in mind to remember. In this case, I think, *Two B's and two C's*—broccoli, Brussels sprouts, cauliflower, and cabbage.

Other types of "mnemonics," or memory-enhancing techniques, include connecting concepts into an absurd story or associating them with strong emotions, such as humor.

A common illustration is shopping lists. If you have six items to buy in the grocery store and don't have a pencil and paper handy, you might link them in this absurd narrative sequence (which you would actually picture in your mind): "The cereal houses a family of bananas, which are drinking their morning coffee, which they spill on their napkins. But the coffee seeps through the napkins and soils their clothes, which now require a good washing with detergent and bleach."

The same sort of absurd associations can help you remember names: "Jack never sits still, much like a jack-in-the-box." (Or "Jack is very calm, completely unlike a jack-in-the-box.") "Susan looks serious—I hope she won't sue me." (Or "Susan seems laid-back—I'm sure she won't sue me.")

There are also some well-known physiologic factors that can impair memory. These include drinking alcohol, failing to get adequate sleep, and experiencing bad stress. The flip side of these points provides us with some simple targeting strategies for enhancing memory at any age: Avoid alcohol. Get plenty of sleep. And take steps to reduce the bad stress in your life.

Finally, don't forget to make good use of written lists, memos, daily diaries, electronic organizers, and the like. The more you commit to paper or to your computer-based appointment schedule, the less you have to carry around in your head.

Sometimes, such as when I'm doing an interview or giving a speech, it makes a better impression if I can operate without notes. But in other situations, I don't hesitate to rely on written reminders because that frees my mind from the need to juggle mnemonics and allows me to think more creatively.

Keep Exercising Your Mind

Keep exercising, both physically and mentally! The more you use your brain to memorize, the more you stimulate those neurotransmitters, synapses, and other chemicals and connections that enhance the mental process.

Also, experts in the aging brain suggest that vigorous exercise—especially endurance activities like jogging—will stimulate mental as well as physical functioning. That was one of the recommendations from researchers at Harvard Medical School, the University of Massachusetts Medical College, and other institutions gathered at a February 25, 1997, conference in Fort Lauderdale ("Staying Sharp: What's New in Brain Research").

Among other things, they advised that to keep mentally sharp, seventy year olds should engage in aerobic exercise at least twenty minutes per day, three to four times a week. Also, they suggested that taking at least 200 to 400 IU of vitamin E per day might help keep the brain in shape. The explanation, which is in line with the arguments I've made in my *Antioxidant Revolution* and elsewhere, is that the vitamin helps neutralize free radicals, or unstable oxygen molecules, which may damage brain cells during the aging process.

This worry about how well our minds are working intensifies as we grow older—yet there's no need to let this concern become one of those fears that overwhelms the facts. Perhaps the best way to think about this issue is to recognize that mental functioning—like lifting, walking, or stretching—is a physically based activity. If you don't use it, you'll lose it. But, barring a genetically based problem or disease like Alzheimer's, if you do exercise your mind just as you exercise the rest of your body, you should be able to retain youthful levels of thinking and creativity—not only through the boomer years, but well beyond them as well.

BEYOND THE BOOMER YEARS: WHAT TO EXPECT IN YOUR SIXTIES AND SEVENTIES

As I mentioned at the beginning of this chapter, the "boomer" age range—including those born from 1946 to 1964—is an arbitrary concept that arises from generalizations in the popular news media, rather than from scientific research. Although the boomer idea is based on chronological age, you should put your primary focus on *biological* (or physiologic) *age*—and on how to recoup those physical, emotional, mental, and spiritual powers that you may have lost in recent years.

If you pursue the targeting principles in this book, which are designed to help you regain the power of youth, you will probably find that even though you may be in your forties, fifties, sixties, or older, you actually feel and operate at a level that is many years younger.

So what can you expect as you move beyond the boomer years? As the following box indicates, you can expect a lot of activity.

Stamina Strategy
How Well Do Men and Women in Their Seventies Respond to Exercise Training?

A group of healthy but untrained men and women, ages seventy to seventy-nine, were assigned at random by University of Florida researchers to one of three groups: 1) an endurance exercise group; 2) a resistance training group; or 3) a control group, which didn't perform any exercise.

According to a 1989 report on the study in the *Journal of Applied Physiology* (Vol. 66, No. 6, pp. 2589–94), the groups undergoing physical training participated in three sessions per week for twenty-six weeks. The resistance-training group did one set of eight to twelve repetitions on ten different Nautilus machines. The endurance group participated in endurance exercises, such as cycling or treadmill walking, at 50 to 70 percent of their maximum heart rate (or oxygen uptake) for forty minutes during the first thirteen weeks of training. During the last thirteen weeks, they increased the intensity of their exercise to 75 to 85 percent of their maximum heart rate.

Participants in the endurance group increased their oxygen uptake during exercise by 16 percent during their first thirteen weeks of training and by a total of 22 percent after the full twenty-six weeks of training. Also, they decreased their heart rate, systolic blood pressure, and "perceived exertion" (subjectively, how tired they felt during exercise). These technical measures are another way of saying that specific endurance training enabled this group to increase their endurance or aerobic capacity significantly.

The resistance-training group didn't experience significant changes in maximum oxygen uptake (personal aerobic endurance) or in their other cardiovascular responses, such as heart rate. But they did increase their lower body strength by 9 percent and their upper body strength by 18 percent.

The researchers concluded that healthy men and women in their seventies can respond positively to prolonged exercise training, with adaptations similar to those of younger individuals.

What this research indicates to me is that if older people are willing to take the necessary steps, they can tap into the power of youth! Also, this study highlights some of the effects of targeting, or specificity training, where a particular kind of activity builds a particular kind of physical capacity. In other words, the endurance group developed more endurance, and the strength group developed more strength.

If you've been doing a good job of identifying your health problems and devising effective targeting strategies, you can expect more of the same—a relatively high level of physical energy, emotional balance, and an optimistic outlook on the future. If you are just starting with your targeting program, you can actually expect to recover some of that vigor and drive you have lost.

In any event, to keep your level of physical functioning and overall stamina high, you'll need to weight your aerobic-strength axis, which we discussed in Chapter 2, more and more toward the strength end of the line. In other words, the strength proportion of your workouts should move toward 50 percent—because one of the greatest dangers you face is the loss of muscle and bone mass due to aging. If you fail to guard against this inevitable deterioration of bodily tissue, you'll pay the price in terms of a declining ability to function physically at youthful levels.

But there's more: you'll recall that aging is also characterized with reduced aerobic power, or endurance capacity. To protect yourself from this danger, you must continue with a rigorous endurance program—even as you step up your strength work.

Finally, don't forget the issue of flexibility. The aging process also involves a steady loss of range of motion in your joints and muscles. This increasing tightness and stiffness can be one of the major threats to your energy levels—and can also result in muscle and ligament tears or other injuries when you find you have to respond to an unexpected physical demand.

In this regard, I'm reminded of a number of sprains, a pulled back, and a hairline fracture that I suffered after I passed age sixty. These occurred during intense physical activity—on a particularly intense training run, a vigorous rock climb, and the ski slopes. In practically every case, I can trace at least part of the problem back to a failure on my part to do sufficient stretching of the injured body parts. The older I become, the more stretching I find I must do if I hope to avoid injury and maintain a youthful physical capacity.

In short, you have the potential to become what I have come to call a "senior powerhouse"—or one of the new breed of older people who are steadily "pushing the envelope" on what it means to retain the power of youth well into old age.

8

. . . .

The New Breed: The Senior Powerhouses

As I move closer to the "Senior Powerhouse" category, I'm often asked about my own exercise routine. Because of the constantly changing demands of the aging process, that's not an easy question to answer.

As I grow older, I find that to minimize the natural deterioration of my muscles and bones, I have to increase the proportion of my activity that I devote to strength work and "striking"-type endurance exercise. Right now, I schedule at least two days a week for strength work, and I'm on the verge of adding an extra day on a regular basis.

Also, because of the inevitable loss of aerobic or cardiovascular power, I have elected to do more endurance work, but at a lower intensity than when I was younger. This means scheduling time at least once a day, seven days a week, for walking, jogging, mountain hiking, biking, or the like.

As for stretching exercise, that's always been a problem with me. Ever since I ran track in college, I've been relatively inflexible, unable to touch my toes from a standing position. That has always bothered me, and I'm especially concerned now, as I begin to push seventy years of age. The older we get, the stiffer we become, and with stiffness comes a reduced range of youthful motion and overall functionality. To remedy this deficiency in my personal fitness, I'm now in the process of adding extra stretching exercises to my daily routine.

In any event, even though my program is certainly not perfect and is constantly under review and being tweaked and adjusted, here is a snapshot of my regimen as this book goes to press.

First, there's my endurance work, which comprises about 65 to 70 percent of my workout. You'll note that this is more than the 55 percent I recommend for people my age—but there's a good reason.

You see, I tend to spend much more time in all types of exercise than the average person. As a result, I feel free to devote much of my "elective" activity to the endurance sports that I love, such as walking with my wife in the cool of the evening in our neighborhood in Dallas, or mountain hiking on picturesque trails near our vacation home in Colorado.

More specifically, I'll try to walk, run, or combine a walking and running routine every day of the week. Typically, on reasonably cool days, I'll run about 2.25 to 3 miles at our Aerobics Center in Dallas at the end of my workday (at about 6:30 P.M.). I'll begin with a slow, half-mile jog (at a rate of 5 to 5.5 miles per hour) to warm up. Then, I'll increase my pace so that for the next mile and a half, I'm moving along at an 8- to 9.5-minute pace per mile. Finally, I'll speed up and finish the last quarter mile in about 2 minutes (an 8-minute-per-mile pace).

On hot days—such as those of 100-plus temperatures we had in Dallas for many weeks in 1998—I'll take it easier. Often, I'll run a half mile, and after that I'll walk for about a minute. Then, I'll run for another half mile.

Most of the time, I'll follow this running routine three to five days a week. Then, the other days I'll walk at home, either a brisk two-mile outing by myself, or a slower two miles with my wife, Millie. More often than not, I'll carry my little dog, Holly, a seven-pound Pekinese, just to make the walk more challenging.

As for my strength training, I devote at least two days a week to sessions of about twenty minutes with weight machines. Mostly, I work on my upper body and back, though I do some quadriceps (thigh) work as well. Strong quadriceps are an especially important factor for me because you have to have strong upper legs for downhill skiing and mountain biking—two of my favorite activities when I'm on vacation in Colorado.

Also, because of the need for extra strength training as I grow older, I'm currently planning to add an extra day of weight work to my regimen. At the present time, I figure I devote 70 percent of my exercise each week to aerobic work, and only 30 percent to strength training. As I've mentioned earlier, this division doesn't bother me too much because I do much more endurance exercise than the average person. If I tried to add enough strength work to make my regimen perfectly balanced for my age—55 percent aerobic and 45 percent strength work—I'd have little time for work and family!

My stretching routine, which I know is inadequate, consists of doing the sleepyhead stretches right after I wake up in the morning. These are described briefly in the example of Diane in Chapter 1, and in more detail in Chapter 2. Also, to clear my head in the early hours, I'll sometimes do twenty or so push-ups.

The last thing at night, I'll use a targeting routine that has proved highly effective in helping me get rid of the tension of the day, including stiffness and spasms that tend to build up throughout my back. This stretching movement is quite simple: I'll lie flat on my back on the floor, and try to straighten my spine out against the floor.

Usually, my back really hurts when I first assume this position. But as I continue to push my back gently against the floor, the tension drains away. After a couple of minutes, I find that I become totally relaxed—though sometimes, as I'm doing this stretch, I have to guard against Holly, who likes to jump on my chest if she sees me stretched out like this on the floor.

When I'm on vacation or away from my regular office routine in Dallas, I'll usually alter my program. For example, when I was on a cruise ship recently in the Baltic Sea, I ran or fast-walked a total of forty miles in two weeks, using a track laid out on the ship. While in Colorado for two weeks during the summer, I'll typically walk briskly two miles in the morning. Then, I may work for a couple of hours, and follow up with a lunchtime break that involves going out for a mountain-biking workout for five or six miles on hilly terrain. Finally, I'll usually walk another two miles with Millie or friends in the evening.

As you can see, I try to vary my routine considerably. For one thing, the variety helps keep more parts of my body in shape through cross-training. For another, engaging in a number of sports keeps my interest up. I'm like anyone else in that I can become bored—and be tempted to cut back on my workouts—if I try to do the same activity day in and day out.

In any event, my fitness program is considerably different from what it was fifteen, twenty, or thirty years ago. And I expect it will continue to change as I age—and as my interests lead me to other conditioning activities.

But now let's quit talking about me and focus on you and your program. What kind of senior powerhouse are you becoming? Here are some of the factors you should keep in mind, depending on your particular health status.

THE SECRET TO BECOMING A SENIOR POWERHOUSE

When you make it into your seventies, you usually face a fork in the road of life—a choice that depends heavily on your previous health history.

If you have already suffered some serious health problem, such as a heart attack, cancer, or the like, you must take the path that involves focusing heavily on reducing the risks associated with your particular condition.

In other words, if you've had problems with clogged arteries that have resulted in a heart attack, you must plug cardiac rehabilitation concerns into your fitness programs. This usually means giving extra weight to a diet low in unsaturated fats and "trans" fatty acids (i.e., hydrogenated fats), going in for more frequent heart function examinations (such as treadmill stress testing, fast CT scanner evaluations, and perhaps arteriography, which are X rays of arteries). Also, you may be placed on a regimen of statin medications.

On the other hand, if you have entered your seventies relatively unscathed—and you've undergone regular medical exams that show your risks of major disease remain low—the chances are you won't have to worry about being surprised by one of the major killers like cardiovascular disease or cancer. So you can take the other path in the fork in the road: one that requires you to "continue to march," with a systematic fitness and diet regimen, and a ready arsenal of targeting strategies to meet the health challenges that will inevitably arise as you age.

As mentioned at the conclusion of the previous chapter, moving into your seventies and beyond requires you to concentrate even more heavily on your strength program. In other words, you should be spending about half your time on exercises that will build your muscles and bones, because your vulnerability to the loss of these tissues becomes an increasing threat as you move toward the outer limits of life. And yes, strength training can include lifting weights as the study in the following box indicates.

Stamina Strategy
Should an Older Woman Pump Iron?

The answer to this question may be yes—and it may be best to go for heavier weights and lower repetitions, according to a July 1996 report in *Clinical Physiology* (Vol. 16, No. 4, pp. 381–92).

Researchers from the Veterans Affairs Medical Center, Palo Alto, California, evaluated a group of sixty-five- to seventy-nine-year-old women, who engaged in fifty-two weeks of resistance training. One group exercised by performing seven repetitions, using resistance equal to 80 percent of the maximum that they could lift in one repetition. Their exercise regimen consisted of three sets of leg presses, knee extensions, and knee flexes, three days per week.

A second exercise group did the same exercises, except that they lifted weights equal to 40 percent of their maximum. The third group was a non-exercising group of controls.

The researchers found that both the exercise groups had significant gains in their thigh muscle strength—59 percent for the high-intensity group, and 41.5 percent for the low-intensity group. Also, the size of their thigh muscles increased. In addition, the bone mineral density of the high-intensity exercisers, who used the heavier weights, increased in the thigh bone.

Even as you focus on strength training, you mustn't neglect your aerobic and flexibility work, because the forward movement of age will endanger those cornerstones of your youth as well.

Sounds exhausting, doesn't it?

In fact, you may question whether or not it's really worth it to devote so much time and energy just to gain a few centimeters of muscle mass or a few points on the bone density scale.

You may decide, "Now that I've made it to my golden years—now that my responsibilities and stresses in life have diminished—I just want to enjoy myself. So I think I'll let up, take it a little easier . . ."

I've heard this litany in one form or another from most of the older people I know, especially when they move into their seventies and approach age eighty. For that matter, I've felt that way myself at times.

But guard against this attitude! Too often, a well-conditioned older athlete begins to let up as he reaches advanced years. Yet inevitably, when an elderly man or woman goes into "retirement" from a conditioning program, deterioration takes over. In a matter of months, if not weeks, it becomes harder to maintain your balance, walk for long distances, and even do simple chores around the home.

One eighty-year-old woman, who had been a regular walker (an hour a day, six days a week), stretcher (seven days a week), and hand-weight user (fifteen minutes a day, four days per week), began to feel some extra aches in her shoulder and also her lower legs. So she dropped her program for a few weeks—"just to take a little rest," she explained.

Unfortunately, her advanced age accelerated the deconditioning process. After only about three weeks, she was hobbling about, feeling her age, and becoming tired after even the simplest tasks.

She actually began to consider suggesting to her children that perhaps the time had arrived for her to enter an assisted living facility—until one of them pointed out there might be a connection between her inactivity and her lack of energy and vigor.

"Before we check out one of these old-age homes, Mom, why don't we try an experiment," her son suggested. "Go back to your exercise routine for a week or so, and let's see if that makes a difference."

The woman objected at first because she felt that physically she just wasn't up to it. But in fact, her physical complaints were the direct result of her having dropped her fitness regimen—a fact that she quickly learned when she tried her son's "experiment." After only about a week, the aches and pains disappeared, her energy started to return, and she was feeling like her relatively young self again.

This scenario is replayed again and again among older people who have discovered that an overall fitness program is the best targeting strategy known to head off the deterioration of aging. (See the two following boxes on leg cramps for examples of such targeting.) But it's necessary for the older person to be vigilant in avoiding the temptation to "take a breather" from a lifelong fitness routine. Remember: Old Man Time is always waiting in the wings, ready to pounce on your muscles, bones, aerobic power, or flexibility—or all of the above—when you decide that you, unlike every other human being, are somehow immune to the ravages of aging.

Quick Fix
Leg Cramps, Part 1: Some Targeting Solutions

Leg cramps, a common problem in the elderly, may be caused by a variety of conditions, including changes in temperature, contractions during electrolyte (body salt) disturbances, medications, and occupation-related factors, such as sitting or standing in one position for much of the day. But as we age, the most common kind of cramp is labeled *idiopathic* by doctors—meaning that the cause is unknown.

Although sometimes no treatment seems to work, physicians and patients have discovered three strategies that may be effective: stretching exercises, quinine sulfate, and vitamin E. (See *American Family Physician*, Nov. 1995; 52[6]: pp. 1794–8.)

Leg Cramps, Part 2: A Case Study

"Margaret," who was in her seventies, was experiencing pains and cramps that reached down the back of her thighs into her lower legs. She had experienced sciatica as a result of a lower back problem that had occurred years before. Both she and her doctor feared the sciatica might recur. But the medications and treatments she had taken for sciatica didn't seem to work with this new onset of cramps and pain. The problem was then diagnosed as idiopathic.

At her doctor's suggestion, she tried quinine sulfate. This over-the-counter medication seemed to work at first. But then the cramps and pains returned, and the physician was reluctant to increase the dosage.

So he advised her to increase her daily intake of vitamin E to 800 IU (she was already taking 400 IU per day), and also to begin to do some stretching exercises. In particular, Margaret concentrated on the lower back exercises I have described as sleepyhead stretches. She did the hamstring stretches as well.

Within a week, her leg cramps and pains disappeared. Her swift recovery seemed to indicate that the stretching routine was the effective treatment.

WHAT IS THE POTENTIAL FOR A SENIOR POWERHOUSE?

The trends toward greater vigor and youthful levels of functioning are definitely up for the senior population. A study by Duke University researchers has shown a steady reduction in the percentage of people over age sixty-five who are classified as disabled. In a March 18, 1997, report in the *Proceedings of the National Academy of Sciences,* the Duke investigators found that in 1982 almost 25 percent of the elderly couldn't perform such common tasks as cooking, bathing, or dressing themselves. But that percentage had dropped by 21.3 percent in 1994.

What was the cause of the improvement? The study leaders said that the reason was most likely better nutrition, hygiene, and medical care. Also, an increasing number of postmenopausal women were taking estrogen therapy, which helps prevent osteoporosis and heart attacks.

I might add that another reason almost certainly has been the growing predilection of older people for exercise. A report released by the National Sporting Goods Association on July 13, 1996, revealed that adult participation had increased by 7.1 percent in seven fitness activities between 1993 and 1995. These included walking, running, swimming, aerobic dance, bicycling, calisthenics, and working out with exercise equipment. Even more significantly, the largest hike in activity, 17 percent, was among those over age sixty-five.

In a related set of findings, more than 43 percent of adults age sixty-five and older were completely sedentary in 1987, according to a September 1995 report from the Behavioral Risk Factor Surveillance System of the Federal Centers for Disease Control and Prevention. But only five years later, in 1992, that number of chronic couch potatoes had dropped to 38.5 percent.

Even more to the point, a February 1998 report from the Yale University School of Medicine focused on disability among 213 men and women, age seventy-two and up. At the beginning of the study, all of the participants needed help with at least one basic activity, such as bathing or dressing. The causes of their disabilities included a variety of problems, such as arthritis, stroke, heart disease, and dementia.

But the study showed that even if you become disabled, you can still bounce back. Within two years, almost 30 percent of the subjects no longer needed any help.

The researchers, who were financed by the National Institute on Aging, were encouraged because their findings showed that elderly people with disabilities have the potential to recover and return to full independence. But they noted that the overwhelming majority of those who recovered were eighty-five or younger: only 3 percent of those who were over eighty-five managed to become independent again. (See *The New York Times,* Feb. 3, 1998, p. B15.)

These efforts to maintain fitness and improve health in other respects are undoubtedly resulting not only in lower rates of disability, but in longer lives as well. The "old-old" category of people above age eighty-five is now the fastest-growing segment of the American population. According to the U.S. Census Bureau, that group grew at a rate of 24.5 percent between 1990 and 1996—with some areas mushrooming even faster. In Florida, for instance, the number of the old-old rose by 36.6 percent during that period.

Furthermore, the proven benefits of exercise among the elderly are multiplying so quickly that even I sometimes have trouble keeping track of the trends. Someone recently called to my attention some findings I had missed from a study done by a research team from the National Institute on Aging and the University of Iowa, and published in the *Journal of the American Medical Association* on March 24, 1994. This three-year investigation, which involved more than eighty-two hundred people age sixty-eight and older, showed that those who engage in regular, moderate activity—such as walking or even working in the yard—are half as likely to develop gastrointestinal hemorrhage as those who are sedentary.

Obviously, this is just one of scores and scores of benefits that even moderate activity can achieve. The advantages can range from the purely health-related, to the cosmetic—as the accompanying box on fatty thighs suggests.

Youth Booster
Weights or Walking—
Which Is Better to Firm Flabby Thighs?

A January 1995 Finnish study, published in the *Journal of Applied Physiology* (Vol. 78, No. 1, pp. 334–40), examined the relative effects of eighteen weeks of intensive strength and endurance training on the legs of a group of women, ages seventy-six to eighty-seven.

The strength-trained group increased the total muscle tissue of the thigh (1.5 percent), quadriceps (4.5 percent), and lower leg muscles (11.2 percent), as compared with a control group that did no exercise.

Also, in comparison with the endurance group, the strength-trained women experienced a significant increase in their quadriceps muscle mass. At the same time, the relative proportion of fat within the quadriceps muscles (which extend across the front of the thighs) decreased. This shift in favor of proportionally more muscle and less fat in the thighs didn't occur with the endurance group.

The investigators concluded that intensive strength training can increase muscle size in elderly women and reduce the relative amount of intramuscular fat—whereas endurance training couldn't accomplish the same result. My observation: there seems to be some evidence here for spot firming, even if not spot reduction, of fatty thighs.

But even though much has been accomplished for the older segments of the population on the fitness and youth-recovery front, much remains to be done. In particular, more older citizens must be convinced of the need to gear up their fitness regimens.

For example, a study published in March 1997 in the *American Journal of Public Health* reported that less than 1 percent of those age seventy-two or older in New Haven, Connecticut, had a normal walking speed of four feet per second. Also, only 7 percent of these senior citizens could walk fast enough to make it across intersections safely before the lights changed.

Here are some other areas related to the health of the "senior powerhouses" that need to be targeted—and if possible, resolved:

Youth Boosters for Retirement

High-powered career people, and especially men, often have trouble adjusting to retirement. Research at Mount Sinai School of Medicine in New York City may have helped to pinpoint the underlying problem.

It seems that men have a natural ability to focus all their energy on one objective—which for most of their lives is their work. So when they stop working, they are often unable to find other meaningful outlets for their energy—and their health suffers as a result.

Women, in contrast, are better able to juggle many emotions and issues, a quality that enables them to retire and make a smoother adjustment to a nonwork environment.

I've noticed these same tendencies among many of the older male and female patients at our clinic. As a result, I've devised a simple targeting strategy for those having problems with retirement:

First, recognize that men about to retire may have trouble with the adjustment. Then, encourage them to get involved in outside activities that can absorb them as thoroughly as their jobs.

Many church groups have succeeded in this effort by helping their older members begin to focus a few years before retirement on their "spiritual gifts"—which involve nonwork, church-related aspirations and abilities, such as Bible teaching or volunteer service to the poor. Often, when an older person becomes as involved in these interests as in his work, the transition to retirement is quite easy.

Strength and Stamina Strategies for the Old-Old

Remember: I cautioned that a serious temptation as we grow older is to let up on all sorts of fitness efforts, including strength work. But the years of training you may put in before your eighties can't be regarded as "money in the bank," which will last for years after you quit working out. The benefits are great as long as you keep exercising, but when you stop putting in the time in the gym or on your rec room floor, those benefits disappear much more quickly than your financial investments.

The only solution to this dilemma is to stay with the program! In fact, I'd say that for those over age eighty-five, probably the two most important activities are first, strength work and second, an endurance activity such as walking, which helps preserve balance.

But if you've already dropped out and are suffering the consequences—or even if you've never been involved in a formal fitness program—don't despair. There is plenty of research that shows no matter how old you are, you can still regain some of that muscle power of youth by starting anew.

Research at the Tufts Center on Aging, for example, has demonstrated that even women in their eighties and nineties can secure tremendous benefits from a strength program. One study involved ten weak nursing-home residents, six women and four men, ranging in age from eighty-six to ninety-six. After participating in strength-training exercises using exercise machines three times a week for eight weeks, these elderly people experienced significant improvements in their strength, balance, and walking speed, according to a June 21, 1998, report in *The New York Times.*

Pick-Me-Ups for Depression

Depression is one of the most devastating emotional problems confronting those in their seventies and older—and the impact can have serious physical consequences as well.

A study reported in the June 3, 1998, issue of the *Journal of the American Medical Association* (Vol. 279, pp. 1720–6) focused on the extent to which symptoms of depression may contribute to decline in the ability to function among those in the seventies and older. Nearly thirteen hundred people, age seventy-one and older, participated in the four-year evaluation.

The researchers found that physical performance deteriorated steadily as the intensity of depression increased. They concluded that those who report depressive symptoms are at higher risk for later physical decline—and that prevention or reduction of depression could play a role in reducing this functional decline.

For some specific targeting strategies for depression, refer to the "Secrets of Stamina" in Chapter 5, especially the strategies involving laughter and advanced spirituality. Also the discussion of depression as an energy sapper in Chapter 3 should be helpful.

An Rx Response for Declining Vision

The problem of deteriorating vision is particularly dangerous for older drivers.

According to an April 7, 1998, report in the *Journal of the American Medical Association,* older drivers who suffer from a reduced field of vision are twice as likely to be involved in an auto-mobile crash as those with good eyesight.

The researchers, who were from the University of Alabama School of Medicine in Birmingham, evaluated the vision of nearly three hundred drivers, ranging in age from fifty-five to eighty-seven. Then, they checked the participants for three years to see if they were involved in vehicle accidents.

They found that those with a field of vision 40 percent or more below normal were 2.2 times as likely to have been involved in an accident than those with better vision.

Possible targeting strategies: the authors of the study suggested that a field of view test might be used by state licensing officials. Until and unless such a test can be mandated, it would be advisable for older drivers to undergo such a test on their own and then seek medical consultation.

Finding an Rx Response for Suicide

The suicide rate among older Americans rose by 9 percent from 1980 to 1992, according to a government report released January 12, 1996, by the Centers for Disease Control and Prevention.

The suicide rate for Americans sixty-five and older was the highest of any age-group. Although Americans in this age range constitute about 13 percent of the population, they account for approximately 20 percent of the suicides.

Suggested targeting strategy: deal more effectively with depression, such as through endurance exercise routines and bodybuilding programs, which have been shown to boost self-esteem among all age-groups. (Also, check the discussions on depression and pessimism in the energy sappers section of Chapter 3.) Introduce the elderly who are most at risk to counseling programs—and keep them away from the assisted suicide movement and its publications.

A Not-So-Quick Fix for Alcoholism

Alcohol abuse is on the rise among elderly Americans, according to a March 13, 1996, report in the *Journal of the American Medical Association.* In fact, the report said, if the rate stays constant, the number of elderly alcoholics will increase by 50 percent between 1970 and the year 2000. Particular problems with alcohol abuse as a person grows older include dangerous interactions of alcoholic drinks with drugs and medications, and an increased risk of serious health consequences, such as cirrhosis of the liver, falls and fractures, vehicle accidents, osteoporosis, alcohol-related dementia, and cardiovascular complications, such as high blood pressure.

Suggested targeting strategy: if you have a personal history of alcoholism, or there has been alcoholism in your family, consider yourself at serious risk. Alcohol abuse can undercut everything else you may be trying to do to regain the power of youth in your life.

An Rx Response for Vitamin D Deficiency

A deficiency of vitamin D—which is probably a major contributor to osteoporosis (bone-thinning) in the elderly—may have reached epidemic proportions, according to many geriatrics experts. Yet some recent studies show that more than half of some groups of elderly Americans are vitamin D deficient.

In a study conducted at Massachusetts General Hospital and published in the March 19, 1998, issue of the *New England Journal of Medicine* (Vol. 338, No. 12, pp. 777–83), researchers found that of 290 patients studied, 164, or 57 percent, were deficient, and 22 percent were severely deficient. The patients ranged in age from eighteen to ninety-five, and even the younger ones were determined to be vitamin D deficient. Specifically, an evaluation of a subgroup of seventy-seven of the patients, who were under the age of sixty-five, revealed that forty-two were deficient.

Suggested targeting strategies: exposure to sunlight can take care of the production of most of the body's vitamin D, but obviously, this approach wasn't working with those in the above study. Generally speaking, the exposure to the sun must be rather direct, and wearing clothing or a sunblock with an SPF rating of 8 or more can prevent any significant vitamin D production. Furthermore, not using sunblock can increase your risk of skin cancer.

Perhaps the best response is to follow the recommended supplement intake of vitamin D, suggested by the Food and Nutrition Board of the Institute of Medicine. These recommendations are as follows: 200 IU daily for those nineteen to fifty years of age; 400 IU daily for fifty-one to seventy year olds; and 600 IU daily for people seventy-one years of age or older.

Because these values may even be too low, I'd suggest this plan: Take the recommended supplement. Add foods, such as milk, with vitamin D fortification. Expose yourself to at least a half hour of sun every day—but do use sunblock. Together, these various steps should ensure that you'll avoid the vitamin D deficiency—and the accompanying threat to bone density—that becomes more and more of a danger as we age.

Most of the suggestions and recommendations in this chapter can be directly applied by those readers in the "senior powerhouse" age range—from about the seventies on up. But in some cases, boomers with elderly parents or relatives will want to absorb these points and help older loved ones apply them. I know I've been in that position a number of times over the years—and many of my boomer-aged patients are involved in advising and guiding their older relatives.

A similar supervisory or advisory approach is often necessary for younger people—especially children and adolescents. In addition, much older individuals may find themselves thrust back into a child-rearing mode: an estimated four million children in the United States are now being raised by their grandparents! For these reasons, I want to say a few words in the following chapter about how to manage the health challenges of childhood and the transition to adulthood.

9
• • • • • • • • • • • •

The Challenge of Childhood and the Transition to Maturity

A forty-one-year-old woman whom I'll call "Andrea" had been a happy child. She came from a loving, intact family and had attended a good college and embarked on a promising career as a marketing specialist with a large retail organization. By the time she was thirty, she had married, and her first child was on the way.

Everything seemed to be going well for Andrea except for one thing. As she was focusing on her career and caring for her family, she completely neglected her health. She had never been athletic or at all interested in physical activity, even in childhood or her teen years. But fortunately, she came from good genetic stock, with no risk factors for cancer or other diseases.

Naturally trim, Andrea had never had to worry about excess weight—until just recently. Also, her heart and cardiovascular system were still benefiting from the protection of her natural stores of estrogen because she hadn't yet gone through menopause. The only thing she seemed to be doing right from the point of view of good health was to try to load up her family's diet with plenty of fruit and vegetables, and to keep their intake of saturated fats as low as possible. But she did have a sweet tooth, and so rich desserts were often a staple at family meals.

Finally, Andrea's lack of a solid, coherent health plan began to take its toll. She had begun to notice when she moved past her fortieth birthday that her energy levels seemed to be lower. She experienced more backaches too. In fact, she had lost a couple of days of work in the past month because of debilitating pains in her lower back.

Perhaps even more important from her point of view, she really sensed she was getting old. She was almost twenty pounds overweight, and she just didn't like the way she looked in the mirror anymore. Her husband didn't seem to mind, perhaps because he was unathletic himself. His main interests were reading, going to concerts, and attending an occasional play. He always said he had married her for her brains, great sense of humor, and vibrant personality, not for some expectation that she might turn into some sort of sportswoman.

But Andrea was becoming more concerned about the way she looked—and the image she was projecting at work and in social gatherings. She knew she had lost some of the zip that had made her such an asset in social situations and in meetings with clients.

To compound her concerns, she noticed that her eleven-year-old daughter was starting to put on some extra pounds, and like her mother, she wasn't at all interested in exercise. Unlike her mother, she wasn't interested in trying to select healthy foods; greasy fast food was her preference.

This antifitness malady also seemed to be affecting her eight-year-old son. He was quite bright and more interested in curling up with a book than playing ball or going for a run. As a result, he was becoming soft and chubby and sedentary, much like his mother and father.

The turning point for Andrea may have been the emotional trauma of passing the symbolic age of forty. Or perhaps it was a real sense that she was in fact losing the energy and vigor that had marked her when she was younger. Or maybe the trigger was her growing concern for the welfare and future of her children and their health. She saw herself in them—and she knew that if they didn't begin to lay the groundwork in childhood for good health and fitness, they would be facing at least the lack of energy she did at her age—and perhaps even worse complications for their health.

Whatever the cause, Andrea decided that something had to be done—namely, a major revolution in her own health habits and those of her family. First, she set about changing her own life. She incorporated many of the targeting concepts and fitness principles discussed in Chapter 2, tackled and eliminated several of the youth drains in Chapter 4, and in general turned her life around. Within a month, she was spending about four hours a week on aerobic exercise, including a walk-jog routine two days and distance swimming on two other days. In addition, she engaged in strength work and stretching about two hours a week at a local gym.

Focusing on herself first was important because that way, when she finally began to suggest some changes in the lives of her children, they couldn't accuse her of trying to get them to do something that she wouldn't do.

The first key in getting a sedentary child started on a more active lifestyle is to make it fun. The second key is to use physical activity to build the child's confidence and self-esteem.

Andrea's son, Bobby, was the easiest challenge. Because he was only eight, his inactive habits weren't too deeply ingrained. It's true that because he had received no training or encouragement at home, he was behind his peers in developing an ability in sports. But the idea of improving his skills appealed to him—and Andrea found a good strategy to help him get started.

To begin with, strength and fitness are of primary importance for athletic performance when a child is young. Later, when he moves into his preteen and teen years, skills become just as important as fitness. But at his current age, Bobby was in a position to do reasonably well on the athletic field if he could get into shape.

So she convinced him to join her during her workouts at the gym and health club, where they had a family membership. She learned from her own reading and from consulting with various trainers that strength training was fine for young children beginning at around age eight or nine. But there were some rules she was told to follow.

One restriction was that Bobby should concentrate on calisthenics or on doing relatively high repetitions with light weights or resistance equipment. (Growing children who engage in heavy-resistance work, including attempts to lift as much as they can for one repetition, risk damaging their epiphyses, or growth plates.)

Also, it was essential that a knowledgeable adult supervise him during his strength workout. Otherwise, he might make mistakes that could injure him. For example, Andrea learned, it was important that sit-ups be performed on a soft surface with knees bent. Otherwise, a back injury might occur. Also, if he used weights or resistance equipment, he had to have an adult guide him every step of the way to protect him from hurting himself.

In addition to Bobby's strength regimen, Andrea made sure that Bobby got involved in a community soccer league and swim team—aerobic activities that helped him build his endurance.

Before the year was out, Bobby's weight was down to normal, his strength and endurance had increased considerably, and his self-confidence was soaring. He was now eager to join his peers for athletic activities and games, and instead of feeling left out, as he had before, he was now one of the first players chosen for teams.

In short, Bobby was building a solid set of habits that would most likely carry over into adulthood. As a result, Andrea could expect that when he reached her age, he would have a much firmer grasp on what it meant to incorporate the power of youth in his life.

As for his sister, she was slower to respond, primarily because she was older and felt more self-conscious about beginning a fitness regimen. But gradually, she came around as well, and even played on some of the girls' intramural athletic teams at her school. Her motivation was that she knew that her excess weight and soft physique didn't fit into the current "hard body" ideal that many of her classmates aspired to. Fortunately, unlike many of her peers, she had no tendency toward eating disorders, such as bulimia or anorexia.

Exercise and wise dieting made much more sense to her—and they provided her with a much sounder, long-term strategy for elevating her self-confidence and self-esteem.

To sum up, then, Andrea and her children learned through practical experience some of the basic principles for launching a child on the road to a lifetime of youthful vigor and fitness. These included:

- Begin aerobic/endurance training at an early age. This should involve an activity that's fun—such as a team sport that involves a considerable amount of running (soccer is one of the best candidates for young children).
- Begin strength training at an early age. As indicated in the example involving Andrea and her children, starting with calisthenics—such as sit-ups, push-ups, and stretching—as early as six or seven years of age is fine. Even light resistance or weight training can be quite helpful beginning as early as ages eight to ten—but be sure that the children are supervised closely during each workout. Also, be certain that they don't attempt to lift heavy weights while they are still growing, and especially that they don't try maximum-weight, one-repetition lifts.
- Educate your children in good nutrition. The various principles advocated for adults in Chapter 6, Chapter 7, and elsewhere apply as much to school-age children as to adults. The important thing is to inculcate good eating habits at an early age.

Energy Pack
A Good Breakfast Equals Energy for Kids

In a 1997 study Danish researchers from the National Institute of Occupation Health, Copenhagen, examined the effect of energy intake at breakfast on school performance the same morning. The parents of ten classes of children at five different schools altered their breakfast routines at home over a period of four straight days. The 195 families in the study were provided with standard breakfasts containing either low- or high-energy foods.

Teachers were instructed to evaluate the performance of the children at school, though they were not informed about the types of breakfasts the kids had eaten.

How did the respective breakfasts fare?

Kids who ate breakfasts that included at least 20 percent of their recommended daily energy intake (calories) did significantly better on voluntary physical endurance and creativity tests than the children who ate the low-energy breakfasts (less than 10 percent of the recommended daily calorie intake).

Also, significantly fewer children who ate the high-energy breakfasts reported feeling bad, and their feelings of hunger were lower during the morning than the kids who ate the low-energy breakfasts. (See *International Journal of Food Science and Nutrition,* Jan. 1997; 48[1]: pp. 5–12.)

If you can get your children started with these three points, they will be well on their way to a fit, healthy, and energetic adulthood. Of course, there are many other concerns that parents need to consider as they are educating their children in the ways of good health—and helping them to develop habits that will reduce their risks to a minimum. A few of these that might serve as a useful checklist for any parent include:

Accidents

Forget freak skiing collisions or sports injuries. The operative words to keep in mind here are *seat belts* and *bicycle helmets.* Within the past decade, the number of deaths of children in car wrecks, bike crashes, and other collisions has declined 26 percent—and these safety devices are a large part of the reason.

Other common causes of child death, according to the National Center for Health Statistics, include suffocation, drowning, and fire.

As a parent, if you train your child to protect himself—and exert regular supervision when you can't count on the child to act on his own—the odds increase considerably that your son or daughter will make it to adulthood with both body and good health habits intact.

Alcohol and Drug Abuse

In most parts of the country, these problems begin in the preteen years and intensify through high school and college.

Alcohol arrests rose by 10 percent and drug arrests by 5 percent on college campuses in 1996, according to a survey released on May 4, 1998, by *The Chronicle of Higher Education.* There may be some slight cause for optimism, however, according to a national survey conducted by the Institute for Social Research at the University of Michigan. This study said that in 1980, 9.5 percent of college students said they abstained from alcohol, while the number had risen to 17 percent in 1996. But that still meant that in 1996, more than four out of five college students were drinking— and some of them drinking so heavily that they died from excessive alcohol ingestion.

One of the problems with alcohol and drug abuse in the home is that many parents, although concerned for their children and horrified by the idea of abuse, actually resign themselves to the inevitability of the problem.

A 1996 poll conducted by the National Center for Addiction and Substance Abuse, based at Columbia University, found that almost half of all parents actually expect their teenage children to use drugs at some point.

The findings were even higher among baby boomers who had either used drugs regularly or experimentally themselves. Specifically, about two-thirds of this group said they expected their kids to get involved in drug use.

What's more, the study found that these boomer parents seem mostly resigned to the prospect of their kids' use of drugs, and they blame everyone but themselves. In allocating responsibility for the problem, most parents blamed the children, the children's friends, or society at large. Few parents pointed the finger of blame at themselves. About 40 percent said they felt they had little influence over whether their teens smoked cigarettes, drank alcohol, or used illegal drugs.

But despite the denial of responsibility, parents must start early educating their children about the dangers of this destructive habit, or the child's risk of substance abuse problems will soar.

Many more problems could be listed—but most parents are aware of what they are. The central message I want to get across here is that you need a plan if you hope to help your child make a successful transition to maturity.

The targeting concept described throughout this book has been designed primarily to help you design your own adult program for recapturing the power of youth. But as you pursue your goals, it's important to remember the young people who are closest to you—and who, in a few years, will be facing the same problems and concerns you are now confronting.

So what better gift could you bestow upon your child than an understanding about how valuable his present youth is—and what steps he needs to take now to ensure that he will retain his vigor and emotional and spiritual health in the future?

Part 3

LIVING LONG AND WELL

10

. . . .

The Outer Limits of Life

If you follow the recommendations sprinkled throughout this book—and you also happen to be blessed with a reasonably good set of genes—what exactly can you expect in the way of a long and productive life?

As the question implies, the answer must be divided into two parts: First, how long might you expect to live? And second, how well can you expect to live?

In other words, we're confronted with a classic quantity-quality dilemma. Most people assume they want a long life. But after they reflect on the point, they will usually add that they want to retain their youthful powers and energy as well. The idea of spending long years in a state of partial or total disability isn't anyone's idea of a happy prospect for the twilight years.

In fact, the future looks increasingly bright on both these factors—the quantity and the quality of life. There are now so many centenarians around that the famous NBC weatherman and wit, Willard Scott—who has made a specialty of recognizing one-hundredth birthdays—can't keep up with the candidates.

By some demographic estimates, there are now approximately fifty thousand centenarians in the United States (double the 1980 figure), and by the year 2030 more than 800,000 Americans will be over one hundred years old. But the picture that's projected is not one of a completely happy, rosy old age: about 30 percent live without disability in their communities, but 45 percent have some sort of disability, and the remaining 25 percent are extremely dependent. (See *The New York Times,* June 22, 1998, p. 1.)

Furthermore, the U.S. Census shows that about 47 percent of those ninety-five and older are in nursing homes. (The number goes down to 22 percent for those eighty-five and older, and 7 percent for those in the seventy-five to eighty-four age-group.)

What can we do to increase the odds that we'll not only live long lives but highly functional lives as well?

Again, following the targeting strategies in the previous pages—beginning with the strike-strengthen-stretch trilogy in Chapter 2—is the best foundation I can think of. But in addition, here are some random factors that have come to my attention as I've studied the lives of older people who retain the power of youth:

- Exercise regularly (i.e., strike, strengthen, stretch).
- Stay at your optimum weight. (Excess weight, especially around the middle and upper body, is associated with higher mortality.)
- Take antioxidants—especially vitamin E. (Recent studies indicate that this vitamin can strengthen the immune system—and the stronger your immunity is as you age, the better your chances of fending off life-threatening diseases.)
- Stay optimistic. (The flip side: a depressed emotional state may hasten death, especially among the very ill, according to a report in the February 23, 1998, issue of the *Archives of Internal Medicine.* In this study of more than thirty-five hundred hospital patients, a depressed mood increased the chances of dying by 13 to 53 percent, depending on how depressed the person was.)
- Stay involved in meaningful work—either professionally or on a volunteer basis.
- Go in for regular, thorough medical exams. As you grow older, you may "outrun" some diseases, such as heart disease and can-

cer. But you still may be blindsided by other problems linked to the natural deterioration of aging, such as kidney failure or immunity problems. But by seeing your doctor regularly, you can head off many of these diseases—or at least identify and treat them at a very early stage.

- Limit alcohol intake.

These are just a few highlights that have emerged as I've considered the lives of those who have managed to push past the biblical norm of seventy to eighty years (Ps. 90:10), and have moved toward the outer biblical age limit of one hundred twenty years mentioned in Genesis 6:3.

Now, here are a few concrete illustrations of different types of people who have made it successfully to an advanced age. Even in these brief references, you'll be able to glean some of the qualities related to longevity that we've been talking about.

Consider, for instance:

- A one-hundred-two-year-old member of a Pennsylvania engineering firm, who still works about twenty hours a week and holds forty patents. He is an expert at his work—and he loves it.
- A ninety-one-year-old female aerobics instructor, who leads fellow members of her Los Angeles retirement home in regular exercise sessions.
- The "world's oldest person," Jeanne Calment of France, until she died recently at age one hundred twenty-one. She was still riding her bike at age one hundred, and lived alone in an apartment until she entered a retirement home at age one hundred ten.
- An eighty-year-old triathlete from St. Petersburg, Florida, who is training for the Ironman in Hawaii. The requirements are a 2.4-mile swim in the Pacific, followed by a 112-mile bike ride, and then a 26.2-mile run.
- A centenarian, who continued to bowl until he was one hundred three and finally died in October 1997 at age one hundred eight.

- Senator John Glenn, who at age seventy-seven is training to go back into orbit as the oldest active astronaut.
- Noel Johnson, perennially the oldest man competing in the New York City Marathon, who pursued a remarkably strenuous training regimen throughout his eighties. He did nine-mile runs three times a week, and after the run, he would work out on a stationary bicycle. Then, he'd do weight training on his "off days." He died in January 1996 at age ninety-five.
- A dozen or so ninety-plus senior tennis players, who participate in the USTA-sponsored Senior/Seniors Tennis Classic in Orlando.

These seniors have varying lifestyles and varying advice about what one must do to live long. But one common thread that jumps out at me is that they all seem to love life. They continue to be involved with activities or work that they love, and people that they enjoy.

Now, take a closer look at yourself. How well do you think you're aging right now? Would you say you're aging well, or not so well? Is the power of youth an integral part of your life, or do you feel that you are losing ground?

Most likely, you have some general feelings about where you stand, but after all, this is a book about specificity training. So it's only appropriate that we get specific in discussing your current sense of exactly how old or young you feel in particular areas of your life.

Here is a practical, down-to-earth quality-of-aging quiz I'd like to leave you with. Just answer the questions—and then you'll see whether or not you need to turn back and reread some of the recommendations and observations we've already covered.

THE QUALITY-OF-AGING QUIZ

Question #1: Can you get in and out of your car easily—or do you find you have to move a little slower than you used to, perhaps to allow stiff muscles a chance to relax?

Question #2: Either sit on a bicycle, or sit at a table and imagine you're on a bicycle. Keep your hands on the "handlebars." Now, turn your head to the right and look to your rear. If a person or car were behind you, could you see it without straining your neck and back?

Try the same movement on the other side by turning your head to the left.

Question #3: Can you carry a packed suitcase as far in the airport without resting as you could when you were twenty years old?

If you don't know, put some heavy books in two equally weighted suitcases and see if you can walk two hundred feet without stopping.

Question #4: Can you carry a heavy bag of groceries as far today as you could when you were twenty?

Question #5: Can you do as many push-ups (or modified push-ups, with knees staying on the floor) without stopping, and bent-leg sit-ups (in sixty seconds) today as you could when you were twenty?

Question #6: Is your sex drive as strong today as it was when you were twenty?

Question #7: Do you laugh as much today as you did when you were twenty?

Question #8: Are your emotions more balanced and tranquil today than when you were twenty?

Question #9: Do you feel you handle stress better or worse today than you did when you were twenty?

Question #10: Do you experience more bad stress today than you did when you were twenty?

Question #11: Are you more optimistic or less optimistic today than at age twenty?

Question #12: Do you have more or less of a sense today that life has a deep, ultimate meaning than you did when you were twenty?

Question #13: Do you have a deeper spiritual life today than you did twenty years ago?

Question #14: Are your personal relationships richer or less rich today than they were twenty years ago?

Question #15: Do you become fatigued more easily today after a hard day of work or a physical outing that demands endurance than you did when you were twenty?

Question #16: Do you look forward to the future with expectations and dreams more or less than you did when you were twenty?

The answers to these questions will be radically different for different people. Also, there is usually no single set of answers that can suggest one person is clearly more youthful, in emotions or body, than the next person.

On the other hand, we can make a few generalizations. For example, if you indicated problems with stiffness in Questions 1 and 2, that certainly reflects the impact of aging and suggests you need to concentrate more on specific stretches that will make you more flexible.

If you indicated a gradual weakening in Questions 3 through 5, that's normal if you haven't been pursuing strength work. If you have been involved in strength training, your loss of muscle power may have declined only slightly, if at all. (In fact, many of my patients who begin a strength-training program in middle age or even later find that they are actually stronger than they were at age twenty!)

Question 6 reflects a normal decline as you age—though as we've seen in previous discussions, regular exercise can certainly strengthen the libido.

As for Question 7, many people tend to get more serious, if not sour, as they age. That's something you can certainly change—though you'll probably have to work on it if you're a "serious" person with "serious" responsibilities in life. A good place to begin is the local video rental store: check out a few comedies and go to sleep with a few laughs on your lips.

Questions 8 through 11 reflect your emotional strengths—and certainly, a sign of successful aging is the ability to marshal your emotions to deal with difficult situations.

Questions 12 and 13 raise the question of your spiritual health. Age should always bring some progress in this area.

Question 14 raises an interesting issue, because many times a person may recall great times with friends when she was younger. But she senses that now, her relationships are more restricted and she is more isolated. If that's the case, it's important to begin to reach out again to others, perhaps by combining a renewed spiritual life with friends who share the same beliefs.

Question 15 is a telltale sign that aerobic power and stamina are slipping away. Yet they can be regained, at least to some degree, through the targeting programs suggested in this book.

Question 16 is in many ways the clincher. When you're in your fifties or sixties, you don't have to harbor dreams about becoming the leader of the free world or winning a Nobel Prize. But you should always be looking forward and sense that you have goals to accomplish—or "fish to fry," as we say in Texas.

Certainly living a long time is a good goal, and maintaining your ability to function at a high physical and mental level into old age is an even better goal. But perhaps the best objective of all is to live a long, active, and richly abundant life. I can imagine worse ways to close out this great adventure and prepare to embark upon the next.

Conclusion

· · · · · · · · · · · · ·

The Power of Youth, the Joy of Age

B eing a "post-boomer" myself, who is still a couple of years shy of age seventy, I find myself approaching that interesting "senior powerhouse" category that I described a few pages back.

Most of my career is behind me, and my chronological youth is certainly long gone. But I still feel significant surges of that power of youth that we've been talking about in this book.

I sense an energy, vigor, and forward-looking optimism that make me want to get up early, work hard all day, and savor a demanding physical workout. I regularly look forward to enjoying my family times in the evening—and more often than not, I want to put off bedtime as long as possible, just to make the day last a little longer.

Of course, I've been blessed in many ways. I've had the privilege of founding and building an internationally recognized preventive medicine health center, which has provided many people with life-enhancing, and sometimes life-saving, health care. My intellect is constantly being stimulated and stretched by bright colleagues, new book projects, and adventures with politicians, scientists, and spiritual leaders in every corner of the world.

There have been problems to be sure: a near-bankruptcy, challenges to my reputation by other physicians, and heavy opposition from my superiors in the military when I was still on active duty with the air force.

The stress has been almost unbearable at times. I tell my friends to look into my face and see the deep furrows and grooves imbedded there. Those lines were earned in hand-to-hand combat on the front lines of many medical and business battlefields.

Over the years I've fought to put the Cooper Aerobics Center, Clinic, and Institute for Aerobics Research on a firm professional and financial footing. I've dueled with opponents on scientific issues ranging from the usefulness of exercise to the value of antioxidants. And I've agonized over whether, or how far, to expand our operations and expertise to other locales and other venues.

I cite these struggles just so you'll understand that I'm not some Pollyanna, talking in a vacuum about the aging process. I've "been there, done that"—and sometimes I've failed miserably in trying to follow some of the principles mentioned in this book.

For example, I haven't always handled bad stress well, and as we've seen, bad stress can be a deadly poison for the power of youth.

But remember: working to regain the fading or lost energy and vigor of an earlier day is a multifaceted process. I may lose my battles with bad stress from time to time. But I have also learned that I can counterbalance this deficiency with a disciplined fitness program.

I may cut my sleep short too often—but I keep working to correct my deficiencies in this area. Guilt can be a great motivator when the cause is true and just!

I stray sometimes from the foods I know I should eat—but usually, I pay close attention to my nutrition. I eat my five to seven helpings of fruit and vegetables each day, including the cruciferous kind (the "two B's and two C's").

I may travel too much and suffer the consequences through too many cases of jet lag. But I'm also quick to take steps to counter the effects of that jet lag, such as the measures described in the youth drain discussion in Chapter 4.

I even skip an occasional workout—and that's a major confession coming from the person who is the source of the definition of "aerobics" for the Oxford dictionary and the *Encyclopaedia Britannica*. But I always feel a pang of remorse because I know I've lost an opportunity, even if ever so slight, to ensure that youthful strength and endurance will remain a vital part of my life as I age.

In short, I know I don't do a perfect job of following my personal power of youth program—and I don't expect you to either. But I have made a commitment, beginning nearly forty years ago and extending in my mind, at least, to the very end of my life, to pursue a basic strike-strengthen-stretch fitness program.

Also, I've developed a number of specific targeting strategies, which are designed to help me overcome special challenges in my life, such as high stress, loss of sleep, and the rigors of travel.

With this combination—a basic fitness program and a set of targeting techniques to help you respond successfully to specific problem areas peculiar to your daily existence—you can't go wrong.

So if you come away from this book with anything, I hope that it is this:

First, design a basic strike-strengthen-stretch fitness program and stick to it, at least three to four times per week. Don't regard it as a short-term affair, but rather as a core commitment that you will keep until you draw your last breath.

Second, analyze your personal energy status right now, as precisely as you possibly can. Identify those specific health concerns and issues that give you the most problems—and are most likely to sap the vigor and joy from your life. The best tool I know to accomplish this is the Cooper Energy Scale, described in Chapter 3.

Finally, be systematic in tackling the particular problems you've identified—and devise a specific targeting strategy to resolve them.

Remember, you've been learning to apply in your ordinary daily life those specificity training principles that are used by elite athletes to maximize their performance. World records don't fall unless someone figures out how to run a little faster or jump a little higher. And the usual method to break through new barriers of achievement is to analyze the problem—take it apart piece by piece—and then devise a specific strategy to solve that problem.

. . . .

For world-class athletes, this means fine-tuning muscle groups, skills, and movements to the sharpest edge. For you, the targeting strategies may seem more mundane—but the results in terms of how well and how long you live can be even more dramatic.

After all, an athlete is called upon to "show his stuff" for only a short time—perhaps a few seconds for a sprinter or high jumper, or a few hours for team athletes or others whose events require more time. But you are dealing not with seconds, minutes, or hours, but an entire lifetime—your lifetime. By becoming an elite player in the game of growing older, you'll not only discover the power of youth, but also a more elusive treasure—a sense of joy in the very process of aging.

Index

About the Author

Kenneth H. Cooper, M.D., M.P.H., is the best-selling author of *Aerobics, Controlling Cholesterol, Dr. Kenneth H. Cooper's Antioxidant Revolution, Faith-Based Fitness, Advanced Nutritional Therapies,* and *Can Stress Heal?* His books have sold more than thirty million copies worldwide. Dr. Cooper coined the term *aerobics* in 1968 and has received worldwide recognition for his contributions to health and fitness. Dr. Cooper lives with his wife and family in Dallas, Texas.